THE NEW MANUAL OF
yoga

KAREN ROSS

ARCO PUBLISHING COMPANY, INC.
NEW YORK

Second U.S. Edition, First Printing

Published by Arco Publishing Company, Inc.
219 Park Avenue South, New York, N.Y. 10003

Library of Congress Catalog Card Number 74-75398
ISBN 0-668-03472-6 (Library Edition)
ISBN 0-668-04347-4 (Paper Edition)

Printed in the United States of America

Contents

Introduction   9

Yoga, the Total Way of Life   13

Yoga Breathing (Pranayama)   20

Relaxation and Self-Awareness   28

Yoga Asanas   36

Advanced Asanas   79

Concentration and Meditation   91

Yoga Hygiene   98

Yoga Diet . . . A New Look at Food   104

Summary of Asanas   112

Foreword

OUR sincere and grateful thanks to Arlene Corwin, (Mrs James Council), a Yogin of some fifteen years standing, for her unfailing help and criticism in the preparation of this book, and for posing for many of the pictures.

Our thanks also to Mr Denis Tannsley for posing at short notice, and a special thank-you to Jennifer Council for showing us all how easy Yoga really is.

Karen Ross
Bruce Perry

Introduction

YOGA is not simply a set of exercises. It is a total way of life for millions of eastern people, and has been so for over 6,000 years. It teaches that a whole man consists equally of body, mind and spirit, all three of which must be fully developed before an individual can realise his full potential. Yoga does not differentiate, as some western philosophies do, between mind, body and spirit, but considers them inseparable.

In presenting this book outlining part of the Yoga systems as being relevant to modern western life (to fully understand Yoga would entail a very full study for a great many years), we do so in full awareness of the fact that many readers may not consider all the Yoga lores and beliefs compatable with our own modern knowledge. But this should not detract in any way from the benefits which such readers may gain from the practice of the asanas (therapeutic postures), and the breathing, relaxing, concentration and meditation exercises.

One does not need to subscribe to the whole of the Yoga philosophy or to follow the complete Yoga Way of Life to enjoy these benefits. The basic principles outlined in the book will show you the way to bodily fitness, to complete bodily and mental relaxation, and to concentration, the better to overcome the problems of every-day life.

Increasingly, business men find that, even if they are not actually suffering from one or more of the tension-induced diseases, they are well on the way towards them, and more and more of them find, when the annual holiday comes round, that they are so in need of complete rest that they spend what should be a period of enjoyable leisure, in a health farm, a retreat house, or even a nursing home.

This is obviously not the better way of life for which we work so hard, and it is quite obvious that the situation will not improve. We live in an age when an executive is considered 'over the hill' at forty-five, and he may well bear out the truth of the inference, since his health may be more than suspect, and he finds it increasingly difficult to clear his mind of hundreds of niggling little worries so that he can think clearly and constructively about the problem in hand. Ideas no longer 'come off the top of his mind', as they did when he was younger, and if he digs deeper, he finds a kind of intellectual chaos which allows him to go no further.

But this is not, of course, a book solely for the business man. Yoga is universal, benefiting all people of all ages. The elderly, for instance, for whom only some of the asanas are suitable, can improve their general health, and maintain their intellectual keenness. The aging process is inhibited, sometimes reversed, as many people, particularly around middle age, find themselves considerably rejuvenated, physically as well as intellectually.

Women who must, by force of circumstances, stay at home, or who do not want a career, but feel restricted and confined within a narrowed life, find Yoga especially helpful, as life takes on new meaning with the revaluation of one's true self and potentiality.

The modern Western civilized individual is both educated and informed as never before. It is virtually impossible for any individual to be unaware of the fact that we ourselves have created the environment and style of life that leads to our own destruction, and that this destruction has already begun, not with the bang of an atomic bomb, but the whimper of the patient in the hospital bed, the sighing of the iron lung, the soft sounds of kidney and heart machines. For every one hospital patient who is the victim of a bacterial disease, there are five who lie in regretful knowledge that if they had lived differently, eaten more wisely, avoided the tensions of their particular life, this would not have happened to them. We are aware of this. We are aware of the fact that we live in a dangerous society, and that we may, any of us, fall victim to these dangers, unless we do something to make ourselves immune from them.

What went wrong with the bright hopes of the Technological Age? Possibly the fact that, in welcoming each scientific advance, we forgot to take a long term view. Did Henry Ford consider the possibility that the universality of the internal combustion engine might result in a world of under-exercised individuals? Did Baird and the other pioneers of television foresee that it would create an entirely new way of life, in which conversation, literature, music and possibly social intercourse would be almost universal casualties? Today's advantages can become the disadvantages of tomorrow, but once change is set in motion, reversal seems almost impossible, and it falls to most of us to live in a world we did not intend to create, or, in watching the creation of it, and failing to see the implications, we simply let it happen, and sometimes applauded.

But few of us can become drop-outs, because few of us live entirely without some responsibility to others. In far too many cases, tension-induced diseases of mind and body make us drop-outs against our will at far too early an age, and we must abdicate our responsibilities under circumstances we bitterly regret.

This is where Yoga comes in. It cannot change the world. There is no Yoga revolution. But it can change every single individual in the world, and that would be revolution indeed. It enables us to create our own personal armour against the adverse aspects of our world, the armour of greatly improved health against disease of any kind, especially against tension-induced diseases, the armour of a tranquil and well-ordered mind, the armour of total physical and mental relaxation, the armour of a new set of values, of the knowledge of our true selves, of our full intellectual capacities.

Yoga does not call you out apart from the world. It helps you to cope with life inside it with a fitter body and a finer mind. It changes you into the essential integral You, the person you were designed to be.

And it requires very little from you in the process. No feats of strength, no Everest to climb, no weights to lift, no memory courses to be undertaken. Just a few minutes of your time each day, a few postures to assume, a few correct deep breaths, a little thought, some small silence. A little disappointing, perhaps, to those who think that high prizes should be hardly won.

But that is Yoga . . . and the rest is up to you.

There are many paths towards the ultimate Yoga ideal. In this book we deal with Hatha Yoga, the attainment of bodily fitness

through Yoga breathing and Yoga asanas, and with the beginnings
of Raja Yoga through concentration and meditation. A short evaluation
of these and the other Yoga paths is given in a later section of the book.

Yoga, the Total Way of Life

LTHOUGH we have, in the first part of this book, selected those Yoga Practices of the greatest immediate benefit to the average Westerner, there is still a great deal that we can learn from the Yoga Way of Life, especially with regard to the various codes of conduct, which, should we choose to follow them, will certainly make us into better individuals, and were they universally adopted, would make the world into a far better place.

Before we discuss these codes, however, it might be as well to learn something about the beliefs of the Eastern Yogins, especially with regard to their religious beliefs, and how they differ from our own. It may be in the mind of some readers that we have picked out certain aspects of a religious way of life with the same impunity as one might pick out raisins from a cake, and that this may not only be a disrespect to the religion concerned, but a contravention of our own.

The Yoga Way of Life is found basically within two religions, Hinduism and Buddhism, simply because these are two of the most populous religions of the East. To be a member of either religion does not presuppose the Yoga Way of Life, the choice of which is entirely voluntary, and is only concerned with the religion itself in the general sense that one's reverence of God is part of the code of conduct, and is observed according to one's creed. Yoga monasticism is an innovation, and is not the general practice. Yoga is very much concerned with the world, and our conduct within it.

The Eastern religions have a concept of God as universal, all powerful and, to us, remote. The idea of a personal saviour is outside the bounds of their belief, and this is why, in the place of the concept of Christ, they have a conception of prophets and teachers who were wholly men, but divinely inspired. Perhaps it is that because they believe in the *totality* of the power of God, that they see the birth and death of a personal saviour as unnecessary, and therefore unlikely, although many of them see the life of Christ as a valuable example, and much of His philosophy as completely sound.

All religions, however primitive, recognise some form of After Life, and the Eastern faiths believe completely in reincarnation of the spirit again and again. There is also a widely held belief that one's conduct in one life dictates the circumstances of one's next appearance on earth. A sincere attempt to live a good life will result in a reincarnation into a better existence. A poorly conducted life, without respect and thought for others, may result in a return to earth as a dog, an ox or even a cockroach. During one's several lives, one progresses towards the ideal individual, to attain a perfect spirit state freed from the need to return to earth again. Thus one achieves Paradise, Heaven, the Happy Hunting Ground, called by different names according to one's religion, and given different dimensions, or is without dimension, and if our paths to this ultimate are different, the goal is the same, and this is possibly the final deciding factor which unites all those who believe in God, even if the methods of reaching this goal often divides us far too sharply.

The Eastern religions do not proselytize. They do not seek converts, and many of them look with some suspicion on those who wish to join their ranks, although, being almost invariably courteous people, they are pleased to answer questions and to discuss the matters of their faith. But since they do not press their beliefs on others, they find nothing strange in a non-believer following what they consider to be the most obvious codes of conduct. In addition, since Yoga is not an essential of any oriental religion, its practice commits us to nothing in the way of belief in that religion, any more than the practice of Freemasonry commit a Christian of any denomination to the beliefs of Ancient Egypt.

If we, as Christians, do not believe in reincarnation, we certainly believe in living to the full, and living it in the best possible way, and if we reject all alien cultures, we reject the best part of what we now value and revere in what we call the British Way of Life. It is worth considering that Christianity was once, to us, an alien culture. During the two World Wars, we did not destroy every Italian painting, or destroy all music whose composer was once cradled in what had become enemy territory. We have absorbed many cultural and philosophical aspects during our existence as a nation, and Yoga, both as culture and philosophy is becoming absorbed into our existence also, to the enormous benefit to us all.

We mentioned in our introduction that there are many Yoga paths leading to the ultimate union with the divine consciousness, (Samadhi), and have discussed Hatha Yoga, and progressed a little way towards Raja Yoga, union by mental control. Without space to discuss the other paths towards Samadhi, we simply list them here, so that you may study further if you are so inclined. The study of Yoga is fascinating to those with a philosophical turn of mind, and may well take the whole of a lifetime.

1] *Jnana Yoga*: union by knowledge
2] *Bhakti Yoga*: union by love
3] *Karma Yoga*: union by service
4] *Mantra Yoga*: union by speech
5] *Hatha Yoga*: union by bodily control
6] *Raja Yoga*: union by mental control

Thus one sees the universality of Yoga, because every individual can achieve the goal by the choice of the path most suited to him. Hatha Yoga and Raja Yoga are the most usually practiced, but one does not necessarily choose one path to the exclusion of others. Many Yogins pursue all paths, in the perfect Yoga life.

No matter which paths of Yoga are followed, there are eight essential practices.

1] *Yama*: abstention from evil
2] *Niyama*: observances
3] *Asanas*: postures
4] *Pranayama*: breath control
5] *Dharana*: concentration
6] *Dhyana*: meditation
7] *Pratyahara*: sense withdrawal
8] *Samadhi*: self realisation

Of these, we will examine two, Yama and Niyama, more closely, because these are concerned with the Yoga rules of conduct.

a) Yamas
1] Non-violence
2] Truth
3] Honesty, integrity
4] Chastity (if this the chosen way of life), or fidelity
5] Forgiveness

Some Gurus teach that the fifth Yama is concerned with not receiving gifts, because the mind of the giver acts upon the mind of the receiver, to destroy his independence. This possibly has reference to begging as an act of humility, practiced by some Yoga sects. The act of forgiveness as the fifth Yama is more relevant to the Western Way of Life.

b) Niyamas
1] Purity, physical, mental and spiritual
2] Contentment, which follows on purity
3] Austerity, which comes with self-mastery
4] Study of scriptures and books of wisdom, in a continuing search for God and truth
5] Worship of God, and the respect of the Gods of other religions.

The decision to follow the complete Way of Life is usually taken early in life, and a young man becomes a pupil (chela) of a teacher or Guru, and learns from him as Saul of Tarsus 'sat at the feet of Gameliel'. This is an apt phrase, as it expresses the reverence which a chela must hold for his Guru. (One can, of course, live the full Yoga life without this early start, especially as so much has been written about all aspects of the Yoga Way of Life. Prominent among later devotees were the Indian Prime Minister Nehru, and Israel's Ben Gourien).

The Chela did not only attend at his Guru's dwelling for daily instruction, but almost invariably lived with him, and since the Guru was likely to be an elderly man, attended to his physical needs, obtaining food and preparing it. The young man learnt about the simple life by actually living it, no matter what his social status before leaving home, and he learnt about service to others by rendering the necessary practical services to his Guru.

Thus Chela and Guru are interdependant, and Chela gains more than philosophical instruction. If he hopes, in his turn, to become a Guru, he is also learning, if he has the required intelligence, how he will instruct his own Chelas in the future, and how he should expect them to behave.

But he is not expected to swallow his Guru's teaching without remark. He is expected to question, discuss, even argue, because this is one way to wisdom, the other being through constant meditation. If this were not so, the Yoga philosophy would not have advanced by a single thought since its inception, and would have little relevance to the present day. No major religion springs up ready born, but changes by the addition of revelation (it being immaterial at this point from what source the revelation is received, except to admit that thought and meditation constitute two of them), and from the first known Yoga writings in the second century, much has been added, and is still being added to today.

The Chela remains with his Guru until he reaches a stage when he himself can recognize true wisdom obtained through meditation, and, as is said in Yogic circles 'his heart becomes his own Guru'. He has, as it were, exhausted the mind of his Guru, and leaves him, possibly to become a Guru himself, possibly to continue his own seeking after wisdom in a location of his own choosing. (To return to Western fiction, the reader may remember 'Black Narcissus' by Rumer Godden, when the Old General's brother returned to the Imperial Palace, not to live within its walls, but to take his place out on the bleak Himalayan hillside, to the distress and perturbation of the nuns who came to live there).

Thus the progress of Yoga continues towards its ideal, defined in the Yoga Sara Sangraha as, 'The silencing of the mind's activities which leads to the complete realisation of the intrinsic nature of the Supreme Being is called Yoga.' Not all Chelas will exceed their Gurus in wisdom and sensitivity, but those who do will have been helped to the limit of their Guru's total Yogic experience. It is as if successions of dedicated people were forming a human chain, passing each new seeker both bodily and mentally to the head of the chain, so that the ultimate individual progresses towards the goal of union with the infinite while still on the earthly plane.

All religions and all philosophies have their lunatic fringes, and it is unfortunate that it is these lunatic fringes which become known outside their natural locations. The death of a Guru who has helped

many Chelas along the path to wisdom makes no headlines in the
western newspapers, while the exploiters of the Yoga way of life,
those who lie on beds of nails or remain buried for forty days are
always of interest to us, if only for their curiosity value.

(There is an exception to this, in that when people whose very names
make news take up some aspect of Yoga, or any other philosophy, the
names of their instructors are suddenly thrown into prominence. As the
behaviour of these famous people, subsequent to their instruction, shows
no startling change, we are inclined to blame either the teacher or the
philosophy, or both, forgetting that often the fault lies with the
individuals. This reaction, however natural, is comparable to expecting
the physical benefits of Yoga simply by reading about them in this
book, without performing a single asana).

The true Yogin deplores the action of the exhibitionists within its
ranks, because Yoga preaches moderation in all things. Once a Yogin
has learnt the complete defeat of pain, he is quite capable of lying
on a bed of nails (bleeding usually being completely inhibited),
of drinking acid, of suspending respiration for the forty days during
which he is buried alive, of holding one arm above his head until it
becomes withered and useless. He is capable of all these things, but he
recognises them as being only one more step achieved along his chosen
path, an exercise completed, another stage reached and passed, and
of academic interest only. It is useful to be able in inhibit pain when
it arises, because pain can intrude upon meditation, but the inhibition
of pain should not become an end in itself, any more than the
achievement of a perfect body by asanas should become an end in
itself. But the exhibitionists are always with us, in all walks of life,
and these feats can coax money from the pockets of tourists, so that
these performances often degenerate simply into a way of making
money, in the same way as children were (and unfortunately still
are), mutilated to make them into objects of pity, the better to beg
successfully. Such individuals are no longer Yogins, and it is unfortunate
that Yoga should be mistakenly identified with them, causing a certain
amount of confusion in the mind of the general public.

Many Yogins become adept in extra sensory preception and occultism,
both of which are believed to be normal human senses lost to the
civilized human. The existence of ESP is now recognized in the west to
the extent that it is now being researched very seriously, even with
regard to its application in warfare (what other department in modern
life would have available funds?) when it is possible for messages to be

sent directly from person to person without the fear of radio interception. It would have its application in the space programme, too, and would make our present telecommunications look unbearably clumsy beside it. To develop these extra senses pre-supposes belief in them within ourselves, which not all of us possess. There are no specific exercises. Development comes through concentration, usually on the centre of the forehead or between the eyebrows, and might, within the scope of this book, be considered one of the Yoga bonuses.

The complete study of the Yoga philosophy lies outside the scope of this book, by reason of its very intricacies, and the thousands of years it has taken to develop. It represents, without doubt, one of the most comprehensive philosophy studies that one can undertake, and virtually all the major books have been translated into English.

If we may recommend one, which does not constitute particularly easy reading, it would be 'Yoga' by Kovoor Behanan PhD, who, born in Travancore, took a degree in Human Relations at Yale University, and returned to India on a Fellowship to study Yoga for two years, not as his forebears might have done as a plan for a complete Yoga life, but to obtain his doctorate in philosophy. Thus he looks at Yoga critically and with detachment and constructive analysis, and successfully bridges the gulf between Western attitudes and the intricacies of the Oriental mind. It is a book of great value to the sincere seeker after the Yoga truths and concepts, but requires study rather than light reading. It is published by Secker and Warburg.

If the implications of Yoga where the Westerner is concerned can be summed up in a few words, we would offer a short verse from the words of Guru Nanak, the founder of the Sikh religion.

> *The world is an ocean, and difficult to cross,*
> *How shall man traverse it?*
>
> *As a lotus in the water remaineth dry,*
> *As also a water fowl in the stream . . .*
> *So by meditating on the Word,*
> *Shalt thou be unaffected by the world.*

Yoga Breathing (Pranayama)

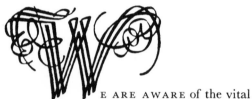

E ARE AWARE of the vital importance of breath, without which we would die within a few minutes, but few of us are willing to face a fact that most of us know, that our breathing is usually inadequate for the body's needs, that we breathe shallowly and lazily, so that the blood is seldom, if ever, sufficiently oxygenated.

The implications of this are more far-reaching than is generally supposed. Many of the vague symptoms of poor health have their root cause in the fact that when blood is insufficiently oxygenated, circulation is slow, and not only are the various internal organs, glands and nerves insufficiently nourished, but the excretory systems do not function efficiently, and the bodily waste products are not removed.

Lack of oxygen is a prime cause of tiredness (yawning is the body's attempt to obtain more oxygen), of brain fatigue and headaches, but in actuality the effects are deeper and more far reaching. Oxygen can be considered the vital fuel of the body, and you cannot run your body at full power on insufficient fuel.

Why do we breathe so badly? Firstly purely from habit, which has engendered a kind of passive laziness, of which we are unaware. Because we feel no breathless discomfort from our shallow breathing, we are not even aware of its shallowness. Secondly, the cramped position so many of us assume during our working days does not predispose to proper breathing, especially if we compress our diaphragms by slumping forward when sitting. Thirdly, our bodies tend to be so stiff that many have actual difficulty in expanding the thoracic cage, so that the portion of the lungs bounded by the ribs is seldom swelled to its full capacity. Fourth, we restrict our breathing by tight and heavy clothes (or did so in childhood, when many bad breathing habits originate). The traditional lounge suit, with a belt around the waistband of the trousers is not conducive to complete breathing, and one sometimes wonders how a woman who wears brassiere and girdle ever manages to breathe at all.

Thus hampered, we breathe in an estimated *one-tenth* of our normal oxygen requirements, and use approximately one-third of our lung capacity. The extremely poor ratio of one tenth to one third is the result of the fact that in addition to only using such a small portion of our lungs, we use that small portion to very poor effect. In fact, the average civilized individual today is not breathing, but merely avoiding suffocation . . . and by a smaller margin than many of us realise.

There are three distinct types of breathing, generated in three distinct parts of the body.

a] *Abdominal breathing*, in which the base of the lungs are filled with air, aided by the lowering of the diaphragm. Men use abdominal breathing automatically, and although it does not represent the whole of the correct breathing picture, it is the most efficient of the three methods, although still inadequate.

b] *Clavicular breathing*, which is natural to women, in which the breath is introduced into the top of the lungs by the raising of the shoulder girdle. It is shallow and inefficient, leaving the rest of the lung static and unused.

c] *Thoracic breathing* is seldom practised unless deep breathing exercises are undertaken, as it involves the raising of the ribs by the dilation of the thoracic cage, and takes a considerable amount of effort. It can best be seen in an animal, a horse or a dog, which uses thoracic breathing during exertion, and is also practiced consciously by athletes.

In Yoga, great stress is laid upon correct and total breathing, and upon breath control. This is called Pranayama, from the Sanskrit words Prana (breath) and ayama (pause), and has come to mean more than mere breath, but also the vital force in every individual.

Pranayama is concerned with more than the beneficial physical effects of correct breathing, since one can change one's mood, especially to establish calm within oneself, by changing the rate of one's respiration. When one is composed and relaxed, one's respiration rate is slow and rhythmical, and when one is excited, respiration rate increases, possibly until we are panting. These emotional states can be created within ourselves simply by the control of our respiration rate, and this enables us to control our emotions to a very great extent, especially to induce calm when we are under stress.

Breathing exercises are performed before each asana session, and before the practices of concentration and meditation, and the first step towards these exercises is to learn to breathe correctly.

It is fairly obvious that, until we become so conversant with Yoga breathing that it becomes quite automatic for us to breath in this fashion, we will maintain two types of breathing, one for our exercises, and one for 'everyday', when we will retrogress into our normal shallow inefficient form of respiration. When from time to time we become aware of our breathing, we will begin to inhale deeply and exhale fully until our attention is distracted, and we forget about it.

And in these conscious moments when we start to breathe deeply, some of us will become aware of a particular problem. Anyone who has paraded under the unsympathetic eye of a drill sergeant, or has attended gymnasium classes, and many who have suffered school PT classes will *automatically* pull in his stomach when inhaling deeply. This may give you an impressively taut military appearance, but it effectively compresses the diaphragm, and prevents air reaching the base of the lungs. To learn to expand the abdomen on inhaling, and to pull it on exhalation seems a reverse of the familiar procedure, and for a while you have to make a *conscious* effort to overcome it. It is often easier to practice your abdominal breathing lying down, until you have developed the new habit.

Normally one sits in one of the Yoga postures to perform breathing exercises, but since one should be as comfortable as possible, it is essential to chose a posture which can be, not only easily assumed, but easily held without strain. There are three traditional postures (also used during concentration and meditation) known as the Perfect Posture, the Lotus Posture and the Easy Posture. In considering the fact that all these three postures are designed to be maintained in

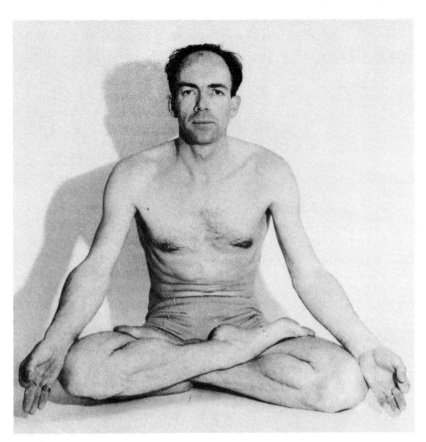

*The performance of the Lotus depends very
largely on the elasticity of the tendons of the hip
joint. Many Westerners never attain it, and
even if it can be performed, it should not be
maintained unless it is perfectly comfortable,
because it is designed to be held through long
periods of meditation.*

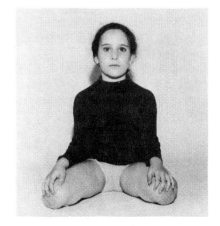

*This position is one normally adopted by
preference by Eastern children when sitting
on the ground, and demonstrates how easily
postures can be learnt if one starts early
enough.*

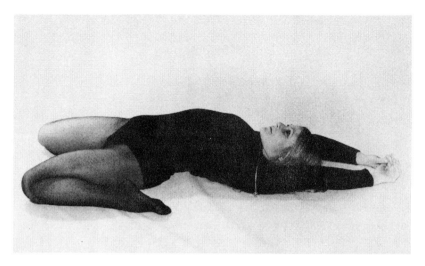

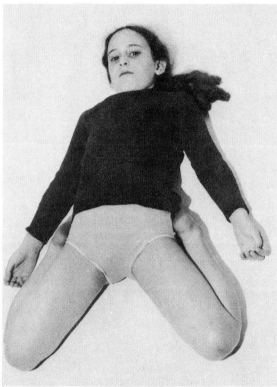

Both Arlene and Jennifer can assume the Supine Pose with ease, the mother because of constant practice, the child through the natural suppleness of the young.

complete immobility for a considerable length of time in perfect comfort, we must also consider the fact that they were designed for Oriental Yogins who, like all Eastern people, squatted on the ground from early childhood. This is not a trait of race, but of environment. In the days of the Raj, the children of officers in the Indian Government Service were usually sent Home to school, and would squat on the floor in the most extraordinary attitudes, often with their legs wide apart and doubled back so that their feet touched the outside of their thighs, and upper and lower legs pressed together, a position impossible for the most athletic English-born child to assume.

This custom of squatting is most probably the outcome of climate. Where the ground is usually dry and hard-baked, chairs and benches are unnecessary, but since the European ground is usually soft and wet, in the absence of something to sit on, a European will stand up and lean against any convenient upright.

Thus the Westerner starts at a disadvantage where the Lotus and Perfect Postures are concerned, and since other postures are quite adequate for the purpose, it is hardly worth practicing and struggling to assume a position which is natural to the Oriental practically from birth. We will therefore consider the Easy Posture, and the Tailor position.

Easy Posture
Sit on the floor with both legs stretched in front of you. Bend your right knee, and place your foot against your left thigh. Bend your left leg and place it under the right. The soles of your feet should, with practice, touch the inside of your thighs.

Tailor Position
If you find the Easy Posture not as easy as it sounds, it is quite permissable to simply sit cross-legged in the Tailor Position, bearing in mind that you should, every day, bring your knees a little further towards the floor. When your legs are supple enough to permit you to sit comfortably with your knees reasonably near the floor, you can try the Easy Posture, but if you wait until you can assume the Easy Posture before you start your breathing exercises and the asanas, you may wait a considerable time before you begin to enjoy the benefits of Hatha Yoga.

Complete Yoga Breathing

Seated comfortably in your chosen position, your hands resting on your knees, inhale completely as follows

1] Inhale into the abdomen by extending the abdominal muscles as far as is comfortably possible.

2] Expand the thoracic cage so that the ribs expand and the chest swells.

3] Raise the clavicles (collar bones) as far as you can without hunching the shoulders.

All this is done in one inhalation, and is done smoothly but progressively, and in the order set out above. You have now filled your lungs completely with air, each section in turn. Exhale slowly.

Once you have established this method of breathing, there are great physical benefits to be gained from learning time control, with the exhalations taking twice as long as the inhalations. There can be a pause between inhalation and exhalation, and the length of the pause will be dictated by the amount of practice you have given yourself. If you start from a ratio of 1:1:2, between inhalation, retention and exhalation, you may gradually work up to a ratio of 1:4:2, but there is no virtue whatsoever in holding your breath with bursting lungs and swimming head, which merely causes discomfort and causes you to exhale too quickly.

An additional breathing exercise . . . practice Yoga breathing first through one nostril and then through the other.

Bellows Breath (Bhastrika)

This exercise will warm the body. It tones up the nervous system and imparts a feeling of well-being and exhilaration.

It consists of a series of very quick inhalations and exhalations, in which one should work, keeping the ratio of 1:2, to make one inhalation and one exhalation in one second, aiding the exhalation with quick inward contractions of the abdominal muscles. The pause comes *after* inhaling and exhaling, and not between inhalation and exhalation, as in normal Yoga breathing. Of course, it may take some time to work down to the time of one second, and at the start it is better to concentrate on the performance of the exercise rather than on timing oneself.

Ten inhalation/exhalation cycles make a very good average exercise. To perform sixty in a minute is possibly the ultimate, and a mark of an experienced adept.

There is another valuable breathing exercise called the Cleansing Breath (Kapalabhati), which is described in the chapter on Yoga Hygiene. It is possibly the most efficient way of clearing the sinuses and nasal passages, and because of its very efficiency, is better performed in the bathroom with a plentiful supply of tissues.

In spite of the insistence on correct postures for breathing exercises, there is, of course, nothing to prevent you from practicing your breathing exercises when standing or even walking. The more often you practice Yoga breathing, the greater the benefit to your health, and it is better to spend waiting moments in correct breathing than in futile boredom or irritation. The beneficial effects of a walk are multiplied a thousand times if you fill your lungs with air and empty them completely, and you will find that, with complete respiration, you will walk faster, will walk further, and will not tire so easily.

You can also, of course, practice Yoga breathing sitting on a chair, provided you hold your spine straight and your head immobile. A few minutes proper breathing while sitting at your desk will clear your head and renew your vigour, and dispel the fatigue of a working day. Even if Yoga breathing in such circumstances is not as totally beneficial as when practiced in a proper posture (which ensures immobility and straightness of the spine) it is obvious that if you wish to cultivate the habit of using the whole of your lungs with every breath you draw, you must practice at every possible opportunity until total Yoga breathing becomes an *automatic* habit.

Relaxation and Self-Awareness

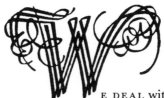 E DEAL with relaxation
before describing the Yoga Asanas because relaxation not only makes
the asanas easier to perform, but also enables us to gain maximum
benefit from them, since they were evolved to be performed with
complete relaxation both of body and mind. Since we relax after each
asana, it is essential that we learn to relax completely and speedily,
and the word 'learn' is used advisedly, because relaxation must be
learnt in the same way as the asanas, and the techniques of
concentration and meditation must be learnt. It is a common mistake
among Westerners to presume, particularly with regard to relaxation
and concentration, that these should come naturally to us, and to
look for some deficiency within ourselves when we find that we cannot
achieve them successfully.

Most of us have, at some time in our lives, made conscious efforts
to relax, possibly with various techniques vaguely based on Yoga
methods, usually with very limited success, or with none at all. The
picture of an individual with furrowed brow and tightened lips trying
to force himself to relax, and failing by reason of the very force he
applies, would be slightly comic if it were not for the fact that he is in
desperate need of relaxation, and defeats himself by his very
desperation.

Bodily relaxation, and the relaxation of the mind learnt in the chapter on concentration and meditation, are among the greatest benefits that Yoga can bestow, because there is hardly an activity, mental or physical, which cannot be better performed under complete relaxation, and hardly a situation which cannot be better met when all tension is dispelled in an instant. If one asks the average Westerner why he considers a knowledge of Yoga desirable, the most probable answer will be 'so that I can relax'.

When we point out that relaxation must be *learnt*, we may seem to be pointing to some far-off goal, and many people come to Yoga for instant help with their immediate problems. We live at a faster pace than the average Oriental, and our forebears were probably living at a faster pace than the founders of Yoga thousands of years ago.

But the paths of Yoga are such that immediate benefit can be gained from the very start of every new discipline, from the first Yoga breath we draw and the first asana we attempt, and from our first studies in relaxation. We do not have to reach a state of perfection to start to enjoy results. It benefits us more to *start* to relax in the proper Yoga fashion than to become mechanically adept in any other type of relaxation exercise ever devised.

This is because Yoga relaxation is complete, relaxing not only muscles, but internal organs, glandular system, lungs, heart, nervous system and *mind*. Other systems tell you to 'make your mind a blank', which is an impossible exercise without further instruction. Yoga is also concerned with the clearing of the mind, but the instructions are explicit, since to do so constitutes as physical an exercise as the relaxation of the muscles.

To perform Yoga relaxation to the full, it is better to have a working knowledge of the structure of your own body, and the position of your muscles and internal organs. Many of us already possess this knowledge, having learnt it at school or in first aid classes, but for those who do not, we recommend a small textbook, obtainable from most libraries, called 'Anatomy and Physiology for Nurses' by Evelyn Pearce.

Relaxation Techniques

1] Assume the Corpse Position, (the ultimate in relaxation) by lying flat on the floor on your back, feet slightly apart, fingers slightly curved. The back of the head should rest easily and naturally on the floor, so that there is no tension in the neck. If this is not comfortable in the early stages, a folded rug or towel can be placed under the neck and under the small of the back. Later you will be able to do without them but, at all stages, complete comfort is essential.

2] Concentrate on relaxing the body muscle by muscle, starting with your toes, one at a time, proceeding from toes to ankle (one leg at a time), from ankle to knee, from knee to hip. Relax the other leg in the same way.

3] Relax the abdomen, and all waist muscles, right round to the spine. Relax the muscles of the chest, of the ribs, of the thoracic spine.

4] Relax the neck, right round, the lower jaw, the face. Relax every muscle of the face, even the tiny ones, smoothing out the frown lines. Imagine your face being made of warm wax, smoothed out without a single wrinkle, perfectly expressionless.

5] Relax the eyes by closing the eyelids very gently, without squeezing. Relax the scalp.

6] Relax the arms, starting with the finger tips and thumbs. Relax each in turn. Relax the hands, wrists, arms, up to and around the shoulders, and then around the shoulder girdle. Relax the back of the neck, the ear muscles, and then the face again.

It is fairly obvious that, as a beginner, you will not be able to achieve total bodily relaxation in one try. You will probably relax your legs, and then, progressing higher, you will find that your legs will tense up again. Your face will constantly become tense with concentration. For this reason, in the early stages, attempt this relaxation process twice at each practice, and remember that even if your muscles only remain completely relaxed for a few seconds, this relaxation, being complete, is beneficial in itself.

Relaxation practices are, at the beginning, rather time-consuming, but as you become more adept this time will shorten and eventually you will be able to relax almost instantaneously, anywhere, and without having to lie down. Obviously, one cannot relax completely in a sitting position, but long train journeys and traffic jams provide excellent opportunities for partial relaxation, and in moments of tension, the ability to perform a lightening relaxation technique is of incalculable benefit.

In the early stages, relaxation may be accompanied by a loss of body heat, and as it is essential to be as comfortable as possible (later

you will be unaware of temperature changes), you can cover yourself
with a light blanket. External circumstances are important only to
the extent that they bother you by impinging on your consciousness,
and if you are bothered by temperature, noise, light or the composition
of the floor on which you lie, you should adjust your surroundings so
that you are aware of them as little as possible. In time they will cease
to bother you, but when first learning relaxation, it is better to avoid
these small distractions. We deal with the matter of dress (or undress)
in the next chapter, and as relaxation commonly proceeds the asanas,
the comments on clothing also apply here.

In relaxing, we become powerfully aware of the Force of Gravity,
and we make use of this in our relaxation techniques. We are, of
course, subject constantly to the Force of Gravity, and although we
combat it with every movement, we are seldom actively aware of it.

Similarly we are seldom aware of our body weight, although we
support it and propel it throughout our waking hours. When we lie
in the Corpse position and begin to relax properly, we become aware
of it, and feel ourselves being dragged down onto the floor by Gravity.
We feel the weight of every limb, of our torso, of our head, which
weighs something like forty pounds. (No wonder the neck is one of the
tensest parts of our tension-ridden bodies.) As we *think* of the weight
of every part of the body, we are at the start of true relaxation.

If you are normally very tense, you may find that, at this point, you
fall asleep. This does not rate as a serious misdemeanour, as it shows
that relaxed sleep is necessary to the body, but if it becomes a habit
you will not progress very far with your exercises because this is only
the beginning of Relaxation and Self-Awareness. If you find yourself
'dropping off', begin the Breathing Technique, which is the next stage
in Relaxation.

Breathing during Relaxation
While you are learning relaxation, your breathing is taking care of
itself, and you have probably been unaware of it. When you have
reached the stage of being able to relax fully and almost automatically,
you will have thought to spare for your breathing, as relaxation
proceeds in its proper order.

Turning your attention to your breathing without changing your
respiration rate is not easy because one tends to quicken the rate.
In hospital, when nurses are taking temperatures and pulse rates,
there is usually a moment when your particular nurse holds your wrist

for what seems an unnatural length of time, apparently looking casually
everywhere but at her patient. She is actually counting your respiration
rate without letting you know, so that it will remain unchanged.

But you must examine your own respiration rate without changing
it, divorcing your analytical self from your physical self. It is
impossible to set out instructions for this in the way that we set out
instructions for the performance of an asana and it is only when
you attempt it that you will find it quite possible, and indeed, easy.

Since you are relaxed and inactive, your oxygen requirements are
minimal, and your breathing will be slower and lighter than when in
action. It should be regular, coming from your Centre of Gravity,
midway between your navel and the base of the sternum (breast bone).
If your breathing is too high, bring it down to its proper place, without
deepening it. If it is irregular, regulate it by *thinking* it into regularity.
(Again this is quite possible in action, even though it seems rather
extraordinary in the reading.)

Now slow the rate of your breathing gradually, still without deepening
it, maintaining the normal inhalation/exhalation ratio of 1 :2.
Relaxation should now be complete, and you should feel a new sense
of bodily warmth, due to the dilation of the blood vessels and the
increased blood flow in the relaxed muscles. So deep is your
relaxation that, should someone lift your arm or leg and let it fall,
you would not feel the impact on the floor.

It is of great benefit to practice these relaxation exercises in bed, as
they will help you to sleep, and, coupled with meditation exercises,
will go a long way to curing chronic insomnia, (which is a habit,
only overcome by the practice of relaxation and meditation for some
time) but to lie completely relaxed is considered to be 85 per cent as
good as healthy sleep, which is a far higher ratio than that obtained by
most insomniacs without the aid of Yoga relaxation.

If you practice pre-sleep relaxation, try to avoid going to sleep on
your back, because your tongue will slip back in your mouth, and tend
to make you snore. This is not only anti-social, but inadvisable, because
you will breathe through your mouth, which is incorrect. Many people
suffer nightmares when sleeping on their backs. Both Orientals and
Westerners normally sleep on their left sides.

Self-Awareness
Self-awareness is an essential part of the relaxation technique, and is
concerned with a reasonable knowledge of one's anatomy and

physiology. It sharpens one's perception of oneself, and is a preliminary to the true understanding of oneself, to self-realisation, without which one cannot reach one's full intellectual and emotional potential.

Thus the path of Yoga runs smoothly, from Yoga breathing to relaxation to self-awareness, to heightened self-awareness through the asanas, to meditation to self-realization, to our true selves in complete control of ourselves, our minds, bodies, and spirits.

Yoga adepts attain control of their internal organs to the extent that they can control, for instance, the beating of their hearts, and can suspend respiration for days on end. But this is a practical book, designed for those who live a practical western life, and we are simply going to explain how the awareness of our own bodies represents a strong bridge between the exercise of complete relaxation and the control of mind. To perform asanas correctly, and to obtain maximum benefit from them, it is a help to know exactly what we are doing with our bodies at any particular stage.

First, we lie relaxed on the floor after performing the whole of the relaxation technique, and proceed as follows.

1) The Outer Layer . . . Skin

a] Think about your skin, which covers the whole of your body, is porous, and yet impermeable to air and water. Think about its elasticity, the protection it affords you, its ability to control body temperature.

b] Start, as in your relaxation exercises, with your feet, feeling in your mind the harder skin on the soles of your feet, the closeness of the two layers of skin between your toes, the sensation of your heels on the floor.

c] Mentally trace the sensation of your skin up your legs, your calves upon the floor, the contrast of the tighter skin over your sharp shin bone, the brush of clothes against your thighs.

d] Continue up your body, concentrating your mind on the feeling of increased warmth, the ridges of cothing, or restricting bands of cloth, of elastic. Feel the contact of skin with skin, and skin with floor. Contrast the feeling of back with floor with heels with floor.

e] Examine mentally each separate finger without moving them, searching for any difference between them. Can you mentally feel difference in length? Does your thumb feel different from your fingers?

f] Make yourself aware of the skin of your face. All parts of your face; cheeks, chin, forehead. Is the skin drier than that of your body? Feel the paper thinness of your eyelids, still without moving. Eyebrows, scalp, again a different kind of skin. Become aware of the difference.

In other words, meet your skin properly for the first time in your life, and become thoroughly acquainted with it, and with its vital importance to you as a sensory organ and your first line of bodily defence.

2) Beneath the Skin . . . Muscles

Obviously few of us have learnt (or having learnt, can remember) every muscle in the human body, for many of them are extremely small and numerous, and the nomenclature is often obscure. But we move finger, toes, limbs, torso and head by moving the muscles concerned, and in this exercise we make ourselves aware of these muscles by actually moving them slightly.

So we start, once again, with our toes, and move each one of them slightly, concentrating, as we do so, on each muscle movement. No single muscle moves in isolation. As we move a foot, we feel the contraction of the calf muscles, a slight knee movement can be felt in the thigh and buttock muscles. Continue your upward exploration, mentally tracing the muscles around the waist, up both chest and back, and into the neck.

When you reach your face, move your jaw from side to side freely. Move your tongue, widen your nostrils, grin broadly. Examine in your mind the muscle relationships in all these actions. *Feel* the muscles work. Frown and then relax, smoothing out the frown lines. Feel how your scalp moves as you frown, and as you raise your eyebrows.

Even if you have no knowledge of the muscles of your body, practice will allow you to become acquainted with them, because you will actually feel them in action. This acquaintance will lead you to control over your body, and over your movements, and will be a great help during asanas.

3) Your Inner Physical Self

Although we do not intend to progress, as Eastern Yogins do, towards the complete control of bodily systems, a certain awareness of our internal organs and physiological processes is a necessary part of the practice of self awareness. Complete bodily control is only learnt after many years of dedicated study, it is started early in life under the direction of a Guru (teacher), and includes the understanding of an Eastern system of physiology which is not always in accordance with our own.

However, a certain amount of physiological knowledge is always a good thing, and helps us to understand the benefits to health bestowed by the practice of our asanas. It also helps us to understand why we should adhere to certain diets, and why such practices as smoking and drinking are inadvisable.

Since we cannot move our internal organs, as we can our muscles, or feel their contact with the floor, as we can with our skin, we must visualize them in their positions within our bodies. (This is where 'Anatomy and Physiology for Nurses', mentioned on page 29 will be of immense help to us.)

Thus we think in turn of our brains (right lobe, left lobe, the point between the eyebrows, the medulla oblongata, where the brain joins the spinal cord), of our senses of hearing and sight, of our lungs (without changing our breathing rate), of our stomachs, liver, gall bladder, pancreas, and intestines, of our bladders, our reproductive organs. Of the glandular system which regulates all bodily processes including that of metabolism. Of the circulation of the blood, of the heart and its action.

All this, at the outset, takes a very long time, but just as, when you become expert, you can practice 'lightening relaxation' without missing out a single part of your body, so you will be able to become totally and consciously aware of every part of the body within a couple of minutes. It is not necessary to practice Self-Awareness every day but, if you do not, you will obviously take longer to reach the speed of perfection.

Yoga Asanas

YOGA ASANAS are not designed to develop muscles, but rather to bring the whole body to the peak of physical perfection and top efficiency by a series of carefully designed positions. Flabby muscles tauten, and assume their proper shape and proportions (excess fat being removed) and women Yogins do not develop a musculature, as can be the case in some other forms of exercise, which is alien to their natural physique.

Those whose muscle structure is undeveloped or under-developed will find that their measurements increase, especially around the chest, but if you seek the enormous biceps and bull neck of the weight lifter, you must look outside the scope of Hatha Yoga.

When we study the table on page 112 we may feel that the claims as to the specific physical benefits of each individual asana must surely be exaggerated, reading as they do rather like those slightly suspect advertisements for patent medicines or exercising appliances seen in the Sunday newspapers. But with 6,000 years on which to draw (and not all research physiologists are 20th century Westerners) there has been time, not only to modify asanas for maximum benefit, but to test the veracity of the claims regarding their physical effects.

If we consider our bodies as working machines we must be aware that those machines are not used by us to maximum advantage. If we consider only three vital factors; breathing, blood circulation, and spinal suppleness, we will see how these factors are affected by our normal daily activities, and how the practice of Hatha Yoga changes them to our benefit.

We cannot be unaware of the fact that we normally breathe inadequately, with the result that, not only do our lungs not expand properly, making us an easy prey to pulmonary conditions and diseases by their very inactivity, but our blood is insufficiently oxygenated, so that every organ and system of the body is poorly (and slowly) supplied with its vital fuel. Blood remains static where it should flow swiftly, and waste products are insufficiently and inefficiently cleared away. If we practiced no other technique than Yoga breathing, the benefit would still be enormous.

The antithesis of a healthy body is not always a diseased body. It is all too often simply a sluggish inefficient machine in which every single system works below par. Were we indeed machines we would be taken down and cleaned, and every part tuned for maximum efficiency. But our very way of life presupposes to our own inefficiency. We sit for endless hours in unnatural cramped positions, increasing the blood congestion in legs and internal organs, bending our heads to create tension in our necks, delaying, by our very posture, the processes of digestion and elimination.

Even those of us who do not have diseased bodies have bodies which by their own inefficiency become easy preys to disease. Except in the case of actual infection (which we are ill-equipped to combat) most of the 'troubles' which send us to the doctor's surgery are the direct outcome of this inefficiency. The defence mechanisms of the body are almost invariably concerned with proper circulation of adequately oxygenated blood, and if you feel this to be too facile an axiom, consider, for instance, the liver, and decide which would be the healthier organ, one which remains congested from years-end to years-end, or the one which is kept in top condition by swift flowing blood, and massaged to stimulate its proper secretion of bile.

Since the blood reaches and nourishes every single part of the body, its effect is total, and when the quality of blood is poor, and circulation is poor, the effects are still total, and the picture is one of general ill-health, or, at best, of being below par. The effects can be felt generally, or both generally or specifically, insofar that one can develop an adverse 'condition' in any part of the body, poor digestion, biliousness, constipation, nervous tension (because nerves also must be nourished by blood) and headaches. Diabetes Mellitus is caused by the inefficient working of the pancreas, and this is often overcome when its efficiency is increased by the internal massage effected by the postures of many asanas. The glands, especially the thyroid gland, suffer greatly from lack of proper blood supply, and the effects are felt, not only in such specifics as skin thickening and loss of hair, and in apparent premature ageing, but in a general lowering of vitality, both mental and physical. The improvement under the practice of Hatha Yoga appears little short of miraculous, and some sufferers of hypothyroidism find that they carr dispense with their dose of thyroxine, simply by the stimulation of the gland by massage, decongestion and increased blood supply. Similarly, many conditions which result specifically from blood congestion, such as haemorrhoids and varicose veins, are greatly relieved by Hatha Yoga, especially in the reverse position asanas, the Shoulder Stand and the Head Stand. But where actual structural damage has occurred, normal treatment should continue and is greatly aided by the practice of the asanas.

Now let us consider the spine, and the fact that almost every Yoga asana seems designed to stretch it in one manner or another. No bony structure in the human body suffers more by the very style of our civilized way of life, and the stiffness which exists in most of us is first caused by our static positions, and then worsened by the fact that, by this very stiffness, any other position becomes painful and difficult to assume. Our intravertebral discs harden and lose their ability to absorb shocks, even the slight shocks that occur in walking, and our spines actually fuse and calcify, and thus, by our own passivity, we abuse our bodies.

The stiffening of the spine is a painless process. We do not feel the development of calcification but the results can be very painful indeed. Nerves and blood vessels become pinched, spinal discs dislodge, and one can stub one's big toe and feel the shock in one's head, since there is no longer anything to absorb it. Muscles weaken, the head bends forward, and shoulders become rounded, cramping the chest. Thus breathing, inadequate to start with, becomes even less adequate, and we are, physically, back where this chapter started. (No single physical system can be considered in isolation, since all are interdependant. Thus inefficiency in one system causes inefficiency in the whole body, but, on the credit side, benefit to any particular system is a benefit to general good health.)

The spine has a tremendous task, not only in keeping the body upright and mobile, but in relation to almost every bodily motion.

All major nerves originate from it, and its effects are far-reaching. Thus a 'slipped disc' in the lumbar region can cause severe pain, possibly as far down as the ankle, which is in itself perfectly healthy, no matter what the sufferer may think. Calcification of the cervical region (the neck) can cause weakening of arms, hands and fingers by the lessening of the blood supply, and of the efficiency of the nerves.

Once our spines becomes supple, and the muscles of the back strengthen, we remove the basic cause of a great number of vague and non-specific backaches which are not the result of disease. Sciatica caused by pinched nerves is often relieved *instantly*, and arthritics often gain new mobility and lessening of pain. Posture is improved, and one feels new strength and vigour.

There are few contra-indications in Yoga, since one never strains to assume a position, and where they exist (they are detailed on page 112) one must use one's own judgement, or that of our doctor. Pain, as opposed to the slight discomfort of the stretching of a long-disused muscle, can be taken as a contra-indication, as can prolonged dizziness beyond the first few attempts at an asana. Commonsense must play a part here. Obviously a sufferer from arterial sclerosis is not going to stand on his head, or a sufferer from spinal tuberculosis bend his spine when pain indicates that he should not. It is as well to have a reasonable knowledge of one's own condition, or to seek the proper advice.

There are some of us who live constantly with pain or disability, and can benefit enormously from the performance of asanas within our capabilities. Many asanas can be performed sitting on a chair, or sufferers can confine themselves to the warming-up exercises, and limit themselves to breathing, concentration and meditation. The Yoga Way of Life is total, and Hatha Yoga is merely a part of it, even if a very important part. If we could only approach Yoga if perfectly fit, we would all remain huddled at our desks with our spines stiffening, our blood congealing in our bodies and our breath growing shorter. If health is a matter of degree, ill-health and disability are matters of degree also, and as we increase the degree of health, ill-health and disability lessens. In all event, as we progress with concentration and meditation, the fact of disability becomes less important even if inevitable. Should we be so totally disabled to the extent that all movement is impossible, we should only be deficient in one-third of ourselves, since we are composed equally of mind, body and spirit, and since most disabilities do not cause a total and absolute loss of movement, our less-than-perfect percentage is likely to be very much lower, and, with judicious use of suitable asanas, almost certain to become even less.

Added Bonuses
One cannot improve our health without having it *show*. Increased blood supply improves the complexion, puts colour in our cheeks, makes the eyes shine, smoothes away wrinkles. A supple spine improves posture and poise, makes us carry our heads proudly, puts spring in our step. We not only delay the natural ageing process, we can, to a certain extent, reverse it. Correct glandular function renews vigour of mind and body. Exercise trims excess fat from our bodies. We feel better, and therefore we look better. This is not a vague hope, but a complete certainty.

Daily Practice ... When and Where
Hatha Yoga is neither a trial of strength nor of endurance, and for this reason it is essential to be as comfortable as possible. This is not merely a concession to Western effeteness, but because one should be as unaware of one's surroundings as possible, since it is not easy to concentrate on one's asanas while over-conscious of heat or cold, of the hardness of the floor, of restrictive clothing, or of the compression of a full stomach.

Location
Ideally (and this means under ideal weather conditions) one should practice out of doors, but since it is more likely that one will have to work indoors, the room should be both warm and well-ventilated. One needs to make maximum use of all the oxygen that one can breathe in, and a stuffy room will soon cause a feeling of tiredness, if not of breathlessness.

The floor should be carpetted, and extra small rugs, cloths such as towels which can be easily folded, or small flat rather hard cushions, should be on hand. To press face, chin, nose or the top of one's head onto bare boards is extremely uncomfortable.

Clothes
The choice of dress (or undress) is purely a matter of personal choice,

only limited by location, since one does not perform one's asanas in the nude in a public meadow, or even in one's back garden. If you prefer to practice privately in the nude, this is entirely a personal matter, although there is a certain amount of personal physical vulnerability which you may care to reduce by protective clothing. Actually, one's reaction to nude yoga can be summed up in one word . . . Ouch!!

The only requirement of clothing is that there should be no restriction of movement, and men usually find themselves most comfortable in boxer shorts *without* a waist belt, and women in jump suits or leotards, or simply in tights and a 'skinny' sweater. Even if you practice your asanas before breakfast, it is not a terribly good idea to wear your underclothes, because the activity engenders a great deal of perspiration, as it is supposed to do.

Timing

There is no fixed time of day for the practice of Hatha Yoga, but you should wait for at least three hours after a meal, two hours after a snack, and until you have emptied your bladder after last drinking. This is not only for the sake of comfort, but because compression may interfere with your digestive and excretory systems while you are performing the actual exercises.

Women who suffer a difficult menstrual period should avoid practice during the first few days. Yoga benefits the reproductive systems and many women will find their menstrual disorders quickly disappear if they practice properly at other times, and that the menstrual cycle is regulated. Abstinence from exercise at this time is a purely personal matter. Some women can carry on their routines without the slightest discomfort, but should go a little easier on the asanas which compress and stretch the abdomen. During pregnancy, it is better to discontinue the ordinary asanas after the fifth month, and practice concentration and meditation only.

Bathing

It is not particularly advisable to take a bath of extreme temperature (very hot or very cold) either before or after exercise because one should start one's asanas at one's normal temperature so that the body has no adjustment to make in this respect and, after the session, one's circulation should be allowed to re-adjust itself in its own time and fashion. A tepid (blood heat) bath or preferably shower can be taken after the asanas are finished, since it will not influence the blood circulation in any way.

Time of Day

The fasting element makes the early morning the best time of day for the performance of asanas if you go out to work (one can take a meal immediately afterwards) with the evening, just before going to bed, a reasonable runner-up. (You can, of course, practice at both times. There is nothing to restrict your Yoga activities to once a day.)

Those who stay at home, especially housewives whose early mornings are taken up with cooking breakfasts and getting the family off to work and school, often find the late afternoon a good time.

Beyond this, as long as the conditions of fasting are observed, one can practice at any convenient time.

Routines

The asanas in this chapter are set out in the order in which they should be performed, and many of them are complementary to, or oppose the following exercise. It is desirable, in the early stages, until suppleness has been achieved, that this order should be followed. If you do not linger over any exercise which may present difficulty (which will be overcome in time by daily practice) you should complete your whole routine in about half an hour, still giving yourself the essential relaxation periods between asanas.

When you become more adept, you will achieve maximum benefit in a shorter time. You may, for instance, prefer to practice the Salute to the Sun which is, as its name suggests, an ideal morning exercise, and can perform some of the quick sets of asanas at odd times during the day. Various asanas can be performed in isolation, to relieve specific conditions such as fatigue, or simply because you feel like it. Rigidity of regimen disappears, and you can use your own judgement and preference in the matter.

Warm-up Exercises

There are three valuable and easy exercises which you can try in odd spare moments, and which help the beginner to 'limber up' before an asana session, especially when one is feeling a little stiff.

1] **Rock and Roll**

Lie on your back, raise your knees, and grip your toes with your
fingers [1]. Rock gently backwards and forwards [2], without going too
far backwards [3] (the nape of the neck should not touch the floor),
until a steady rhythm is obtained. This exercise is invigorating, and
curiously consoling in times of stress, probably because this rocking
motion is the primitive action in the expression of grief.

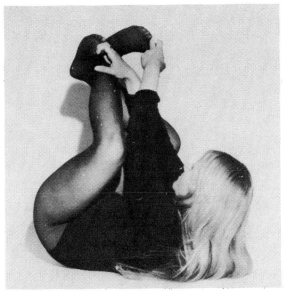

1

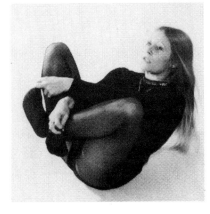

2

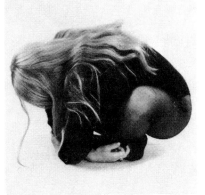

3

2] **The Pump**

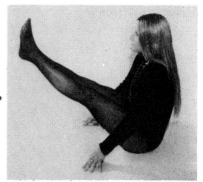

Sit on the floor, hands by your sides, and raise both feet together a few inches off the ground [1]. Without raising legs further swing them together to the side, inhaling the breath at the same time [2].

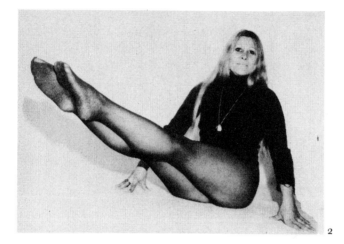

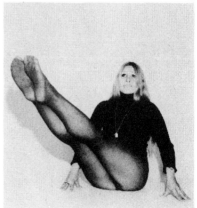

Swing legs as high as possible, and hold them briefly, exhaling the breath [3]. Return to the centre and repeat on the other side. Six movements in all, three on each side, will be found to be quite adequate. Commonly known as the 'Gut Buster', this exercise increases suppleness and strength in hips and thighs, and helps create a neat rear-end.

3] Head Rolling

Possibly no part of our anatomy suffers more from tension and stiffness than our necks, and although they get plenty of exercise during asanas, this is an exercise which can be done in odd moments (traffic jams perhaps) with extreme benefit to our general health. It is a great help in relieving tension headaches.

The human neck is designed to move as smoothly as if on ball bearings (actually it terminates in a peg around which the 'ring' at the base of our skulls lies in the same way as a hoop-la ring lies around the stick after a successful throw) but often calcification and arthritic deposits are such that one can actually hear a gritting sound as we move our necks. These are *not* contra-indications, and perseverance will improve the condition to the extent that they disappear completely.

Let the head fall forward [1]. Inhale and raise the head. Turn the head as far as possible to the right [2]. Tension should be felt in the muscles of the left side of the neck. Count five, exhale, and turn head to the centre.

Repeat, turning head to the left.

Allow the head to droop back by its own weight [3], and then lower

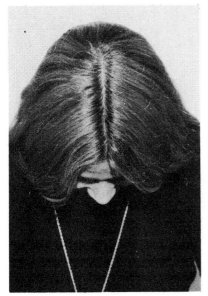

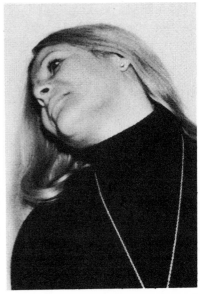

1
2

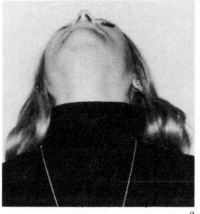
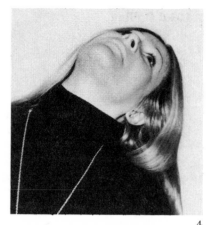

3 4

it to your chest. Now inhale, and while holding the breath, roll the head right round, with your neck held as high as possible [4]. Let it roll by its own weight, your face downwards on the forward roll, as if your body ended at the neck, and the head simply an added dead weight. Roll first from right to left, and then in the opposite direction, exhaling as the head comes to rest on your chest. Repeat three or four times each way, or until neck tension is removed.

Do not approach these exercises, or the asanas that follow, in a spirit of grim determination, because, to Westerners, determination is always allied with tension. Hatha Yoga is surprisingly easy, whatever impressions the illustrations may give. The photographs are often 'action shots', and few of the positions have to be held except in specified Static Phases. Many of the actions during ordinary daily movement would look equally difficult if photographed in the same way.

Naturally, if skill in performance is to be gained in minimum time, daily practice is necessary . . . this is only commonsense, but reluctant or hurried practice does not confer maximum benefits. The discipline of Yoga is purely self-discipline, and if you prefer to forgo a few daily sessions, or to exercise at odd moments instead of at a regular time, the only criticism will be your own. Yoga asanas are meant to be enjoyed, and we must approach them according to our different temperaments, and it is unnecessary to point out that we must interpret the basic instructions in this chapter in the light of our own abilities and physical capacity.

■ The Shoulder Stand/*Sarvangasana*

The Shoulder Stand seems, on first approach, to be a rather acrobatic exercise for a first asana, but, as in all asanas, the method of assuming the position is far easier than it looks in the illustrations, and one progresses in a slow steady movement that ensures correct balance at all times.

There is an Easy Shoulder Stand for beginners who don't have the immediate confidence to go all the way up without a little preliminary practice. Although a fall is virtually impossible, it is quite permissable to perform the asana within a few inches of a wall, but not to lean or push against it in any stage of the asana. It acts as a psychological prop rather than a physical one, and can be dispensed with in the second or third asana session.

The human spine is not intended to be straight, but has natural curves resembling an elongated S, the natural in-curves being at the nape of the neck and just above the pelvis in the lumbar region. The degree of curvature varies from individual to individual, and the lumbar curve is often so pronounced that it is impossible for the spine to be completely flattened against the floor when lying flat on the back. Since one lies flat on one's back at the start of the Shoulder Stand for complete spinal support, those who still have a hollow in the 'small of the back' should slip a folded cloth under this arch, or raise their knees a little, as shown in Figure 2. To leave the lumbar arch unsupported will throw undue and unnecessary strain on the lumbar vertebrae and intravertibral discs. As your Yoga sessions continue, your spine will become more supple, and undue curvature will correct itself considerably.

Starting Position [1]
Lie flat on your back, feet together, arms by your sides, hands relaxed. Tuck in your chin. Relax all muscles, particularly leg muscles.

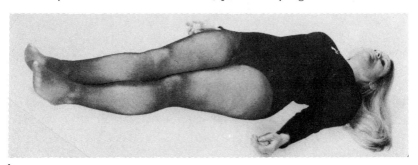

1

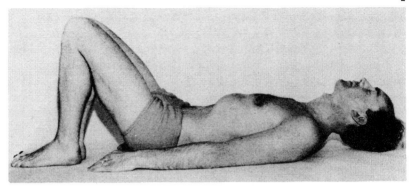

Easy Starting Position (For use when lumbar vertebrae do not touch the floor.) [2] After assuming the normal starting position, draw in the feet slightly along the floor, so that the whole of the spine is supported.

Keeping the whole of the spine pressed to the floor, slowly raise the legs, feet together, *without pointing toes* [3]. (This would create tension in the legs.) Relax all muscles except abdominal muscles, which will be involved in subsequent movements.

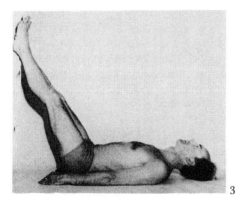

3

Breathing Normal.

Statics You are going to move your legs through a 90 degree arc in this part of the asana, so that they finish at right angles to the floor. Pause twice during this process, at 30 degrees and 60 degrees . . . one third and two thirds of the way through the movement.

Duration Pause for between one and five respirations, according to degree of expertise achieved.

Your legs are now at right angles to the floor, spine fully pressed down, and chin tucked in [4].

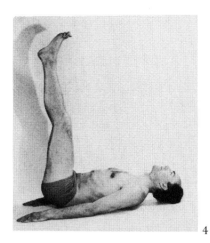

4

Contract the abdominal muscles to assist the raising of the buttocks from the floor. Make sure the back of your head remains pressed down. Raise the legs vertically over your head [5].

Breathing Calm and steady.

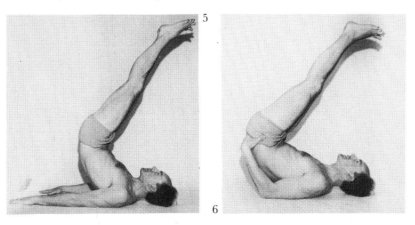

5

6

Variation for Beginners If you cannot raise your buttocks easily from this position, assist the lift by putting your hands around the backs of your hips [6].

Move the legs slowly in a line as nearly parallel to the floor as possible, so that your spine rises at right angles to the floor, and the nape of your neck presses itself down flat [7]. Avoid pointing your toes, so that your leg muscles are properly relaxed. Keep feet together, as at all times in this exercise.

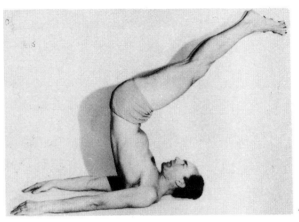

7

Breathing This position will push up your sternum to touch your chin, and may make you feel that you want to hold your breath. Breathing should continue normally.

Concentration should be on easy steady movement, and on relaxation, and this concentration should be carried into the Dynamic Phase.

Final position Contracting the abdominal muscles, raise the legs vertically to their highest possible extent, the trunk following [8]. Do not tense feet or legs.

Breathing Breathe freely.

Static Phase Remain in this upright reverse position as long as comfortable, while relaxing as many muscles as possible. The full beneficial effects will only be felt if relaxation is as complete as is compatable with the maintainance of the position.

Concentration during the Static Phase should be on relaxation, immobility and breathing, which should still be perfectly normal.

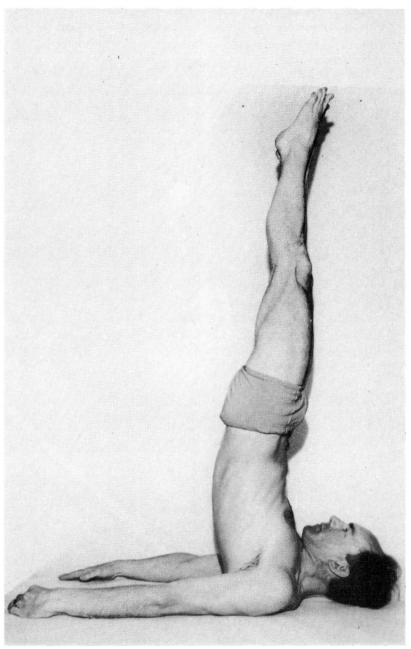

Easy Final Position This is called the Half-Shoulder Stand [9], or Ardha-Sarvangasana, and is easier for those with overweight or other physical problems. Instead of making the full lift after the legs are in the vertical position, bend the lower legs back onto your thighs (the back being supported by the hands), and then slowly lift the legs towards the final upright position. If this lift is practiced daily, the correct final position will be accomplished in a surprisingly short time.

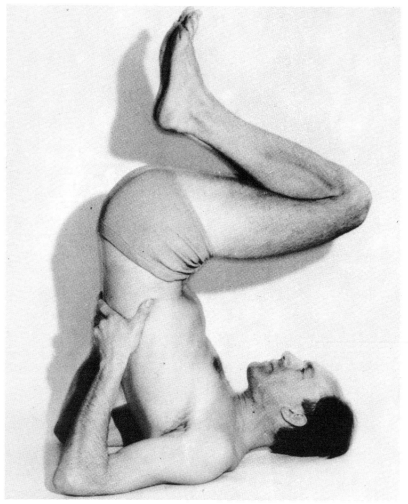

9

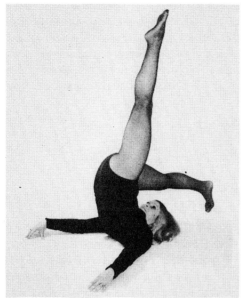

10

Dynamic Phase (Stage One)

From the final Shoulder Stand position, allow first one leg and then
the other to fall to the floor behind your head by reason of their own
weight, assuming the Plough position [10]. (This is actually excellent
exercise for the Plough Asana.) Do not hold the position, but return
to the upright final position without pause.

Breathing Normal throughout.

Return to Starting Position It is essential that you should return
slowly to the starting position, by completing all the movements
by which you assumed the position, in reverse order, and omitting
the Static Phase.

1] Remove your hands from their supporting position. Move legs down
slightly towards their vertical position.

2] Lower spine towards floor and move legs until they are at right
angles to the ground. Your spine should *uncoil*, and not bump down.

3] Lower legs gradually to the ground.

4] Rest

■ The Plough/*Halasana*

This asana is so named because the body in its final position resembled the primitive Eastern plough. This is an excellent exercise for the spine, and for spinal nerves and muscles, and for the thyroid gland. It revives and revitalizes, and dispels fatigue. The final position, as in the case of the Shoulder Stand, is not nearly as alarming as it looks, and is actually reasonably easy.

Starting Positions Both the normal and easy starting positions are identical with those of the Shoulder Stand, and therefore need not be illustrated again. Thus, you once again lie flat on your back, feet together, arms by your sides, palms downwards. (For the Easy Starting Position, draw in your feet a little to flatten the curve in your back, or support the curve with a folded cloth.) Raise your legs until they are at right angles to the floor.

Contract the abdominal muscles so that the thighs rise naturally against your chest, and the base of the spinal column rises from the floor. Keep the legs straight, feet together. Do not point the toes.

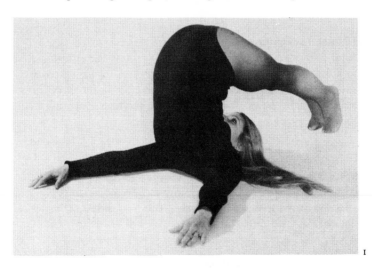

I

Stretch out your legs and allow your toes to touch the floor as far as possible from your head [1]. The greater the distance, the greater the spinal curve . . . and the greater the benefit. If your toes do not touch the floor immediately, do not force them down. They will reach the floor by their own weight.

Breathing Throughout the exercise, breathe normally.

Static Phase (Part One) Having reached this position, hold it for a minimum of five respirations.

Concentration Concentrate on breathing normally throughout the exercise. (Beginners tend to hold their breath.) Concentrate on the stillness required during the static phase.

Final position [2] (not to be attempted until the normal position can be held for the length of ten respirations.)

1] Bend the knees and bring them to the ground on each side of the head.
2] Slide your hands over the backs of your knees, and under the nape of your neck, one hand at a time. (This is not physically difficult, but there is a certain art in balancing which must be learnt.)
3] Push the elbows apart and towards the ground, to increase the spinal arch.

Breathing Breathe deeply to increase the internal massaging effect of the position.

Static Phase (Part Two) This position is, curiously enough, quite a comfortable one to hold, but it must be held in complete immobility, which is psychologically difficult for a beginner. Thus the duration of this immobility must be left as a matter of personal choice.

Concentration Concentrate on your spinal column in its present position, on the thyroid gland in your neck, on the massaging of your internal organs by your position, and your breathing.

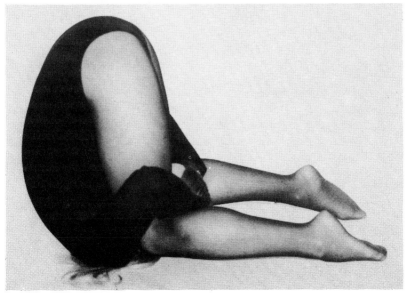

2

▉ The Fish/*Matsyasana*

This asana is so named, not because the Yogin assumes a fish-like attitude, but because, when the lungs are inflated, one is able to float in water for as long as one holds the position, without any further activity. (The experiment is worth trying.)

The asana is the exact opposite of the Plough, insofar that it arches the spine backwards after it has been bent forward, and in fact, all physical implications are reversed. Its beneficial effect upon the thoracic region, and therefore upon your lung capacity, can be seen by the fact that a far greater chest expansion is possible after only a few weeks of practicing this asana.

The Fish is not always an easy position to assume at the beginning, simply because many people tend to be round-shouldered, and where spinal stiffness exists, it most often exists in its upper regions. However, this asana corrects these conditions, and one progresses day by day in the easy Yoga way without strain, reaching a little further in each session, the actual small attempts start to alleviate the conditions, and make final success not only inevitable, but easy.

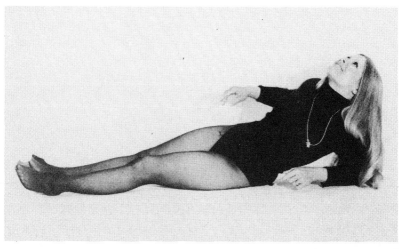

1

Starting Position Sit on the floor, with your legs out in front of you. Leaning sideways, place first one elbow on the ground, and then the other [1]. (If you put your elbows down together, a nasty bruise will be the slightest injury that you receive.)

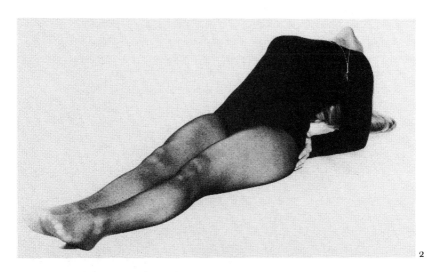

2

Hollow the small of your back by pushing your chest forward, and pushing on your elbows. Let your head fall back to its upmost extent. Keep your buttocks on the floor [2].

Now your head rests on the floor, and the nape of your neck is included in the arch. Your body still receives support from your elbows, which should be moved forward [3].

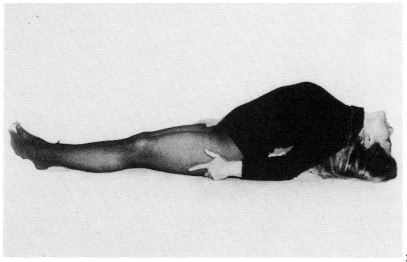

3

Breathing, which should have been clavicular up to this point, should now become full and deep, and abdominal respiration should be reduced. If you can raise your shoulders when breathing, this will ensure the correct breathing in the top third of your lungs, and contraction of your abdominal muscles will empty your lungs completely at the end of every expiration.

Continue this breathing throughout the assumption of the final position.

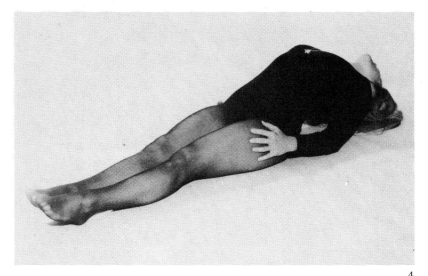

4

Final Position The hands are placed on the thighs, so that the elbow support is removed [4]. It is not easy to maintain the position without their support, but the increased benefit is enormous. This final position should not be attempted until you are accustomed to the performance of the rest of the asana. This position should ultimately be held for the duration of ten deep respirations, and one should work gradually towards this end.

Return Unlike most asanas, the return is not affected by a reversal of the movements, but by simply relaxing the back so that you lie flat on the floor. Rest in this position for a few minutes.

Concentration On clavicular breathing, on the possibility of floating endlessly on water.

■ The Forward Bend/*Pashchimottasana*

This is another spinal asana, designed to exercise, stretch and tone up the lumbar spine. (It is considered complementary to the Plough, which performs these functions for the upper spine.) As in all stretching and arching exercises, it tones muscles and nerves, and greatly benefits the muscles of the abdomen, and the internal organs.

Starting Position Lie on your back, and stretch out your arms beyond your head, so that you lie in a straight line from finger tips to toes (the latter, as in all asanas, should not be pointed). Move your arms up slowly from their position until they are at right angles to the floor, your thumbs hooked together [1].

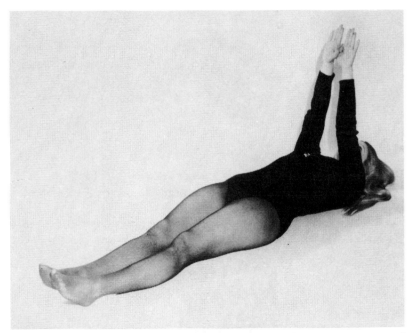

1

Continue to bring your arms down slowly without bending them, lifting your head up at the same time. When your arms form an angle of 45 degrees with the floor, only your head is raised, your shoulders still remaining down [2].

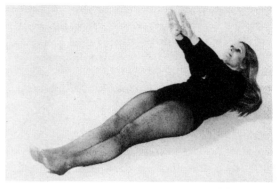

2

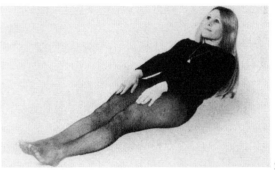

3

The position of your hands dictates the position of your back. As your hands reach your thighs, your back has begun to curve off the ground [3].

The sliding of your hands along your shins completes the spinal curve, which should be as round as possible [4].

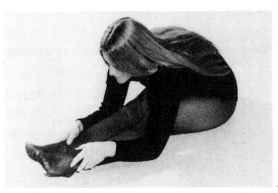

4

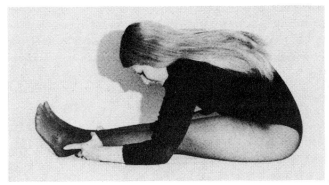

5

Bringing your head down towards your knees makes it possible for you to slide your hands towards your feet [5].
Lowering your forehead to touch your knees [6] may not be possible at your first few attempts, but will become easy as your spine becomes more supple.

Breathing, which should be normal throughout the earlier stages of the asana, now may become a little difficult, because, once your forehead is on your knees, you will find it easier to breathe out than in. You can convert this fact to obtain maximum benefit from the asana if, while still inhaling normally, you exhale completely every time.

Final position Hook your middle fingers around your big toes, and link your thumbs together, pressing your legs to the floor. Your lower spine is now fully stretched.

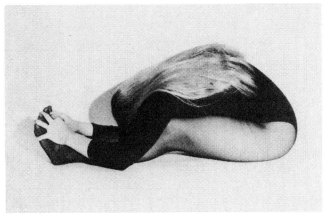

6

Return in reverse order, first by unlinking your hands from your toes, and drawing your arms back until your elbows rest on the floor level with your knees. Lift your head, forehead still parallel with the floor, and replace your hands upon your legs, sliding them backwards so that your spine curls down upon the floor. Begin to raise your arms with shoulders still off the floor, lowering them when your arms are vertical. Lower your head to the floor as your arms reach a vertical position, and then continue the arc until your arms lie on the floor behind your head.

Static Phase After the Dynamic Phase, which consists of repeating the asana and the return three times, there are two Static Phases.

Part One This is a continuation beyond the normal final stage, when the arms are pushed back along the outside of the thighs, and the knees are grasped by the thumb on the knee cap, and the fingers underneath. Contract the abdominal muscles to increase the curvature, and tighten the whole position . . . forehead to knees, face to chest, elbows to sides.

Duration Hold during five deep respirations.

Part Two Releasing the knees, slide the hands along the shins until you can hold your toes. Maintaining this position without bending your knees, pull on your toes to bring your chest down towards your knees, and, with the help of your abdominal muscles, arch your spine to its fullest extent.

Duration Hold for up to ten deep breaths. Five is a reasonable minimum.

Concentration During the Dynamic Phase (the performance of the asanas and return three times), concentrate on the smoothness of your movements, on the separation of each individual vertebra from its neighbours, on the relaxation of back muscles, on breathing.

During the Static Phase, concentrate on the effect of the asana on the base of the spine, not only vertebrally, but with regard to the blood and nerve supply.

■ The Cobra/*Bhujangasana*

The Cobra, another spinal-stretch exercise, is without parallel in removing rigidity, and again imparts flexibility to the thorax. It is an easy exercise, but is a little tricky, because in no other asana is the beginner so prone to make mistakes.

This is partly because its very simplicity, especially in illustration, leads one to believe that attention to detail is not essential, and also possibly because it appears to resemble the 'press-up' found in a number of physical culture exercise. If you are familiar with 'press-ups', you will have to pay particular attention to the instructions, or you may find yourself automatically going into the press-up technique.

Starting Position Lying prone, with face pressed on the floor, feet together, bring your elbows close to your body, hands flat on the floor beside your shoulder [1]. The correct positioning of the hands is very important. The tips of the fingers should be level with the top of the shoulder, and in this case, a fraction of an inch will make a great deal of difference.

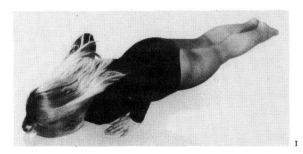

I

The face is carefully pushed forward to stretch the neck *before* it is lifted so that the chin rests on the floor [2]. Neck tension as the chin lifts is an indication that the stretching has been adequate.

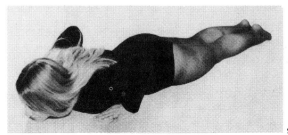

2

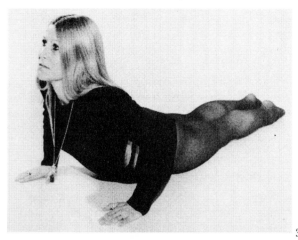

3

The body is raised very slowly solely by the contraction of neck and back muscles, as no pressure whatsoever must be placed on the hands [3]. (If they are correctly positioned, no effective pressure can be placed on them unless the arms are straightened, which is not correct.) When the muscles are fully contracted, maximum rise has been reached. [4]. This rise, of course, improves with practice. Looking up as far as possible helps this rise, but the head should not be thrown back at this stage. The arms still remain relaxed, and no pressure is put upon them. The back will experience a warm flush, and the skin will actually redden, as circulation increases.

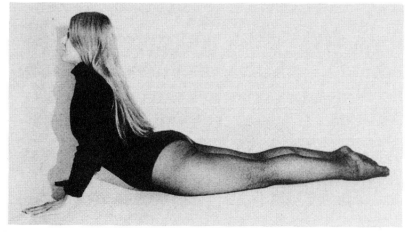

4

Dynamic Phase The last three illustrations demonstrate the Dynamic Phase of the Cobra, which is repeated three times.

Breathing should be normal throughout. Even though you only rest your full face on the floor fractionally, rest it lightly so that your nose is free for breathing, and not squashed into the carpet.

Static Phase Straighten your arms, and push back with them as far as possible, to accentuate the spinal curve [5]. Legs should be relaxed, and feet slightly apart.

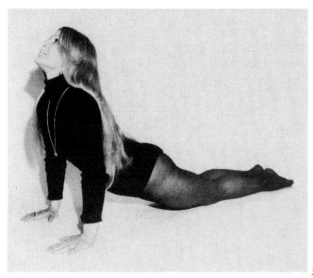

5

Duration Try to start with a minimum of three breaths, and work gradually up to ten.

Breathing During the Static Phase, the breathing is usually reduced by the stretching of the abdomen. You will have to breathe deeply to overcome this.

Concentration *During the Dynamic Phase* on the actions of your movements on your spinal column, on the opening of spaces between the vertebrae, and the release of pinched nerves and blood vessels. *During the Static Phase* On the construction of the spine itself, on the vertebrae, the spinal cord, the elaborations of the spinal circulatory and nervous systems.

■ The Locust/*Shalabhasana*

The Locust is an easy asana to perform, but its beneficial effects are considerably reduced if it is not performed correctly. (Its very ease of performance tends to encourage one to rush through it in a slapdash fashion.) As an asana, it is concerned more with movement than with immobility. In addition to increasing spinal suppleness and blood circulation, it is without parallel in its action on the nervous system. The Locust complements the Cobra, which is why it follows after it.

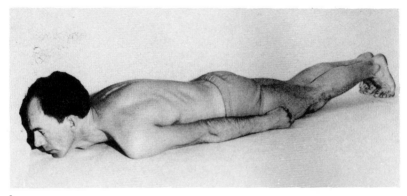

1

2

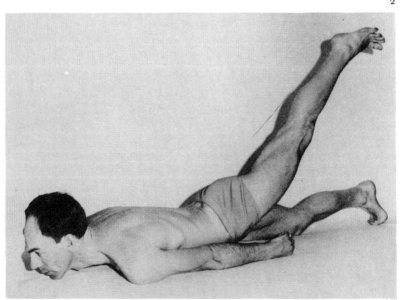

Starting Position Lie face downwards on the floor, legs together,
arms by the sides, hands tightly clenched. Stretch the neck out,
as for the Cobra, but rest the chin on the floor, and not the face [1].
Contract the muscles of the back so that you lift one leg at a time [2].
The movement must come *only* from this contraction, and complete
relaxation of the calf muscles will ensure that this is so. Keep legs
straight at the knee, and press the abdomen onto floor to avoid any
pelvic twist. This position is known as the Half-Locust . . . Ardha-
Shalabhasana.

Final Position
In performing the Complete Locust, the fists are clenched to provide
added power. Both legs are raised together, and are followed by the
raising of the hips, by means of the contraction of the back muscles
alone [3]. Note that the toes are *not* pointed, as this creates tension
in the calf muscles. While the head and shoulders must remain on the
ground in the correct performance of the exercise, beginners may find
that they need to raise them slightly to gain sufficient impetus for the
movement. This tendency must be corrected gradually in further
exercises, or it will lead to the use of this method, rather than to the
reliance on muscle contraction.

3

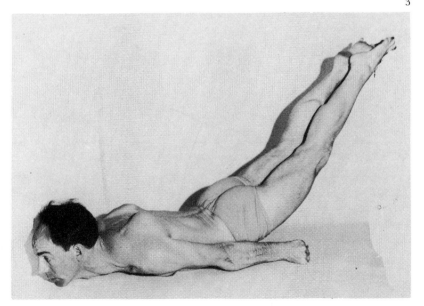

Variation on Final Position This position varies from the previous one only in the position of the arms. The palms of the hands form an arch, instead of being tightly clenched, and are drawn slightly forward [4]. When assuming the position, pressure is applied to the hands to assist the lift (but not at the expense of the muscle contractions), and the head and shoulders remain on the floor. Other variants are shown in the chapter on Advanced Asanas.

Breathing should be normal throughout. It is not always easy to breathe normally during the performance of the Locust, but it should be practiced, and tendency to breath holding discouraged.

Concentration On the correct contraction of the back muscles.

Static Phase There is no true Static Phase in the performance of the Locust, a pause of a few seconds, (not exceeding five) being the limit at the end of both the Half and Full Locust. Relax completely before progressing to the next exercise.

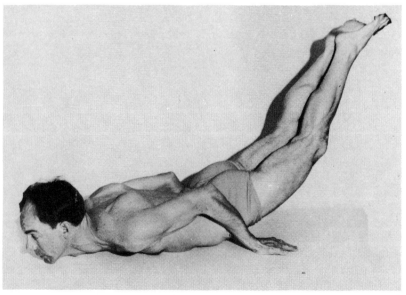

4

■ The Bow/*Dhanurasana*

The Bow represents another backward spinal stretch exercise, and is the antithesis of the Cobra and Locust, insofar that muscles which were active in those two asanas are now inactive, and vice versa. Because of its position, with the abdomen on the floor, the internal organs are massaged and decongested with great general benefit.

The Asana includes one of the most important Dynamic Phases in Yoga.

I

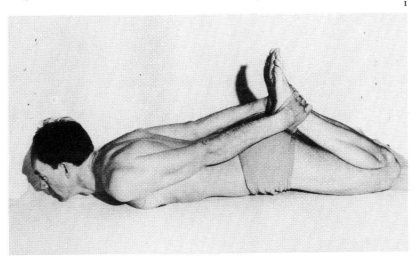

Starting Position Lie flat on the floor, arms along your sides. Relax the back muscles completely, or you will get nowhere. Raise your chin, and grasp your ankles (one at a time until you become adept at it), by cupping *all* your fingers and your thumb over your ankle bone [1]. Part your knees slightly, but your big toes and the inside lines of your feet must touch.

Push your feet back and up in one movement, so that your pubic region leaves the ground [2]. Your knees should be as high as the top of your head. Thus your arms are roughly parallel with your raised thighs, and your torso with your legs, forming the lines of a square. Your arms should be straight, knees apart, big toes together.

Dynamic Phase This consists simply of rocking backwards and forwards in this position, and it will take some practice before any appreciable movement is achieved. Finally you will be able to rock

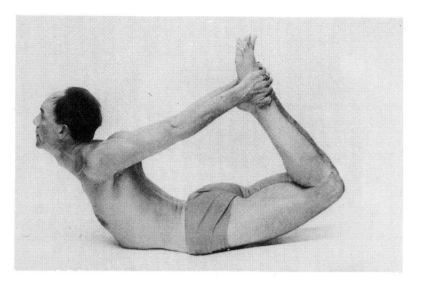

fully, until both chest and thighs touch the ground in their turn. Continue rocking movements until breathless, not exceeding twelve, even when expert. These need not be continuous. It is quite permissable to rest and relax after a few rocking movements, and then to assume the position again.

Breathing You may either breathe normally throughout, or practice inhalation as the head comes up, and exhaling as it comes down. Or vary the breathing procedures during different attempts at this asana.

Concentration On back and abdominal muscles.

Static Phase Immobility in full Bow position for the duration of from five to ten normal respirations, or for as long as possible without strain.

Breathing Normal.

Concentration On complete relaxation of back muscles, especially if the Static Phase follows the Dynamic Phase, during which some tension will have built up.

Return Slowly in reverse order . . . feet to buttocks, knees to floor, arms to side. Relax.

■ The Twist/*Matsyendrasana*

Because the original asana is extremely difficult for Westerners, we normally perform the Half-Twist or Ardha-Matsyendrasana. In previous asanas we have bent the spine both forward and backwards, but now we are going to actually *twist* it in perfect safety, and to stretch spinal muscles and ligaments to their full extent, with the resulting beneficial increase in blood supply. We will also tone up those parts of the nervous system not reached, or imperfectly reached, in previous asanas. We will also improve the mobility of the lumbar and sacral spine, and prevent the calcification which causes stiffness, and finally complete immobility in this region.

This asana is far easier than it looks in the illustrations. Since this is a twist, there is obviously a left twist and a right twist, the performance of *both* being the completed asana.

Starting Position Sit on the floor, legs stretched together out in front of you. Bend the right knee and place your right foot *outside* the left leg, so that your ankle-bone touches the outside of the left knee, and your right foot lies parallel to your left leg, the sole of your foot on the ground. Support yourself on your right arm, which is moved back slightly, palm of the hand flat on the floor. Your left arm should be bent, your hand on your knee [1].

1

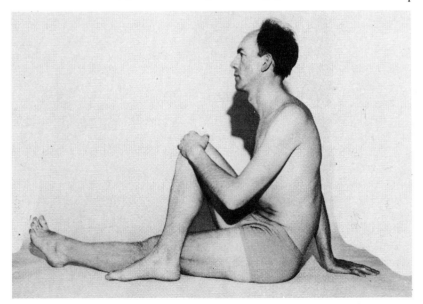

Slide the left hand down to touch your left shin, or, if possible, to grasp your *right* foot [2]. (To grasp the left foot would constitute a simple forward bend, and would not form a twist.) Ideally, the right knee should be almost in your left arm pit, and you should work towards this. The twist should be continued by thrusting from the right arm, the hand of which rests on the floor behind your back. The twist is completed by turning the head as far as possible to the right.

2

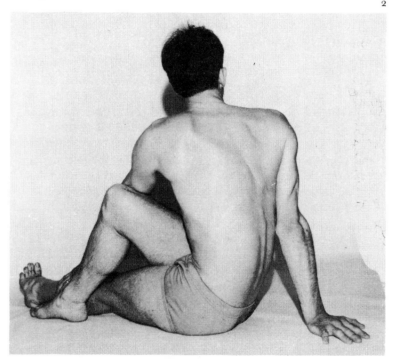

Final Position [3] The right arm is moved behind the back so that it lies across it at the waist, the back of the hand against you [4], and the index finger on the inside of the right thigh.

This constitutes, of course, only one half of the asana, it should be repeated with the opposing twist, starting with the *left* leg being moved across the right.

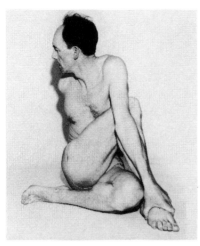

An alternative version of the Twist, in which the left leg, instead of being extended, is kept doubled throughout the asana

3

Breathing Normal, and the position held for between five and ten breathes for each twist.

Concentration on the relaxation of spinal muscles, and on the implications of the spinal twist throughout its entire length, ending with the twisting of the cervical vertebrae as you turn your head.

Two alternative final versions of the Twist, very suitable for beginners who find it difficult to reach down to grasp the foot.

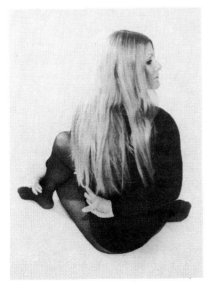

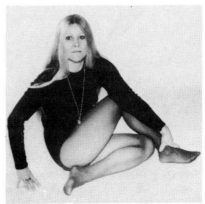

■ The Head Stand/*Shirsasana*

The chief difference between the Head Stand and the Shoulder Stand is that in the Head Stand, the neck is not compressed, so that the whole of the spine is upright in its natural curves, and the blood has free access to the brain, which is normally starved of circulation.

As in the Shoulder Stand, the internal organs are efficiently decongested to their benefit. The techniques of deep breathing assist this decongestion by gentle internal massage. The reverse position of the lungs enables exhalation to be absolutely complete, which, among other benefits, helps to prevent tuberculosis and other lung complaints, caused because the base of our lungs usually remain static.

The spine, especially where intravertebral discs are at risk, benefits greatly from the release of its normal load, and each vertebra regains its normal position with regard to its fellows. Neither spine nor neck are at any risk during this asana, as the neck assumes a natural protected position within the shoulder girdle.

But the greatest benefit in the Head Stand is to the brain, which, by its very position, is the organ least sufficiently supplied with blood. Only when the brain is adequately nourished can one realise one's full intellectual potential, and those of us who suffer periodic 'brain fag', or find difficulty in work of which we feel we should be capable (or of which we have been capable in the past), may often find the solution in renewed blood supply by the practice of this asana.

Those who fear a 'rush of the blood to the brain' need not worry. One does not throw oneself into the childhood 'handstand', but assumes the position calmly, and the valvular system of our circulation precludes a flood of blood to any part of the body, in the same way as a system of locks prevents sudden and widespread flooding of river land with an abrupt increase in the volume of water.

Once you have learnt the easy trick of balance, you will be able to maintain the Head Stand for an almost indefinite length of time in complete comfort. Three minutes is a good average to aim for, and you can perform the asanas as an isolated exercise as often as you like during the day.

Because you are going to have the top of your head on the floor, the weight of your entire body upon it, you will be more comfortable, in the early stages, if you have an additional folded rug under your head.

Starting Position Kneel down on the floor, and place your clasped hands on the floor in front of you [1]. Your elbows should be close to your sides, and your arms should form an equilateral triangle with your body. (If your elbows are too far out, you will throw unnecessary strain on your neck.)

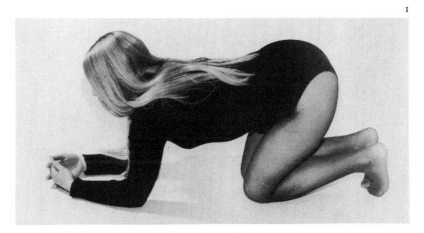

1

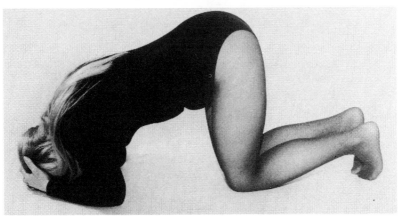

2

Place the *top* of your head on the floor within the triangle of your arms, and the hands, fingers loosely entwined, will help to hold your head steady [2].
Straighten your legs, keeping them together, taking as much weight as possible on your head, which should still be in the same position,
top of the cranium to the floor [3]. Bring your feet as far in as possible without losing balance [4].

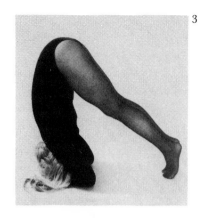
3

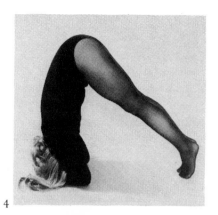
4

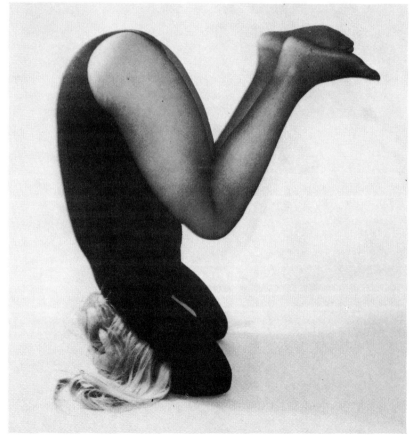
5

Bend your legs, bringing your feet up against your thighs, and your knees against your chest, which should maintain your balance perfectly. Keeping your body perfectly straight and still, raise the legs up in a slow controlled movement [5]. Practice will enable you to find your correct centre of gravity, which will enable you to hold the position comfortably and for considerable periods of time [7].

Smoothness of movement as the legs start their upward movement ensures correct balance during this stage of the asana.

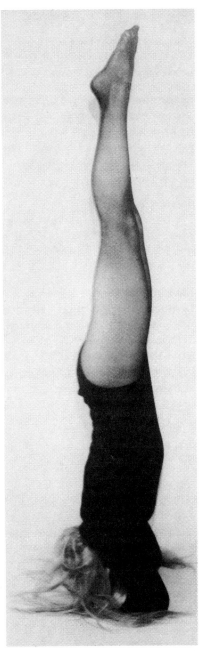

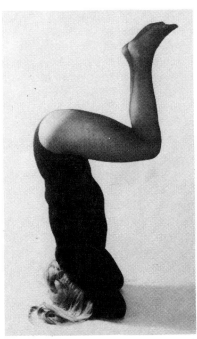

6

7

Breathing Normal throughout.

Concentration Few beginnners meet with instant success when first attempting the Head Stand, and it may be as well to analyse what can go wrong, and how to overcome it.

Dizziness Some people experience dizziness on first placing their heads on the floor in assuming the starting position. This can be overcome by a] practicing a few warm-up exercises, and/or b] straightening the legs, as in the second position, and 'walking forward' with head down and back rounded until the dizziness ceases. Sit up and relax before proceeding.

Somersaulting
If you somersault in the early stages, your neck and back are not straight enough. Possibly you are too stiff and round-shouldered to straighten them sufficiently, and should practice the Cobra and the Bow until flexible enough to try again.

Lack of Balance
If you feel that you must flail your legs or fall, you are incorrectly positioned or you are trying to move too fast. Slow continuous movement is necessary if you are to progress smoothly. Hold in your mind the thought that it is virtually impossible to *fall*, that imminent loss of balance merely means an earlier return to the ground by a series of movements the reverse of those made in assuming the position.

Rest Position
After assuming the Head Stand and returning to the ground, it is desirable to assume the position illustrated below for about half a minute or longer, while normal circulation is restored [8].

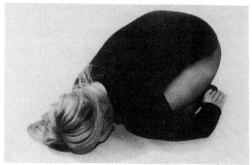

8

Advanced Asanas

NE CANNOT become even reasonably adept at Hatha Yoga in a week or a month. The importance of correct performance lies not only in the final posture, but in the ease and fluidity with which that posture is assumed. It is for this reason that we have separated certain variations of the asanas already described in the previous chapter, and not because they are particularly difficult, although some are a little more exacting than those you have previously practiced.

Because Yogins are not engaged in a race against others who wish to obtain benefit from Hatha Yoga, or training for a contest, there is no virtue whatsoever in straining one's physical capacity at any time by maintaining a stance beyond the limits of comfort, or holding one's breath until one's head swims. Lengthy static and dynamic phases come with practice, and bring their own particular benefits, but concentration during asanas is not only an important adjunct to each asana, but an actual part of it, (correct concentration actually aids us in assuming a position, and in maintaining it), and if we are physically strained beyond comfortable limits, concentration becomes difficult, if not impossible.

Therefore it will readily be seen that it is more important to become adept at the simpler forms of the asanas before progressing to the more advanced than to hurry through to those in this chapter for no other reason than to find out if you can do them. (Patience is one of the many Yoga virtues.)

■ Advanced Shoulder Stand/*Sarvangasana*

This differs from the simple Shoulder Stand insofar that you start
by lying on your back on the floor with your arms stretched out above
your head, as in the Forward Bend (*Paschimottanasana*) and the arms
remain in this position throughout the exercise.

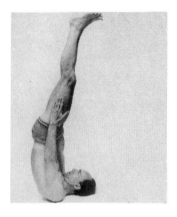

Advanced Plough/*Halasana*

The advanced variations are concerned with the final static phase.
After the bending of the knees to rest on each side of the head, the
knees are not grasped to keep them in position, neither is the nape of
the neck supported by the hands, as the arms are stretched out on the
floor, as shown in illustration [1].

1

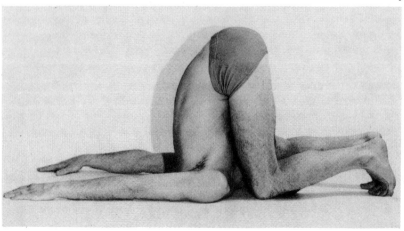

For the performance of this variation, the asana starts with the Yogin having his hands folded behind the head. Proceeding, except in this respect, as for the simple asana, the usual final phase is omitted, and the asana finishes with the legs above the head, and the feet on the floor stretched out as far as possible [2]. The elbows must not be raised at any time during the exercise. This is more difficult than it looks, as there is a great deal of tension in the back of the neck, and the simple exercise and the first variant must be practiced until the neck is strengthened before this is attempted.

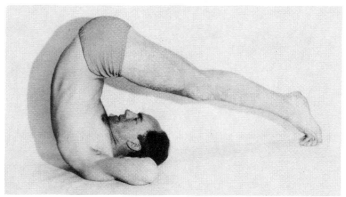

2

■ **The Fish**/*Matsyasana*
The advanced Fish Position starts from the Lotus posture, which most Westerners cannot assume. There is little virtue in struggling to assume a position which is natural to Orientals from childhood, and should the Lotus be impossible for you, the alternative is to assume the ordinary cross legged Tailor Position.

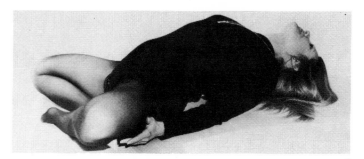

3

■ The Forward Bend/*Pashchimottasana*

The muscular action (and therefore the benefit), of the Forward Bend
is considerably increased if it is performed with the legs apart, instead
of together. The feet are turned slightly inwards throughout the
performance. In the final position, the forehead touches the floor.

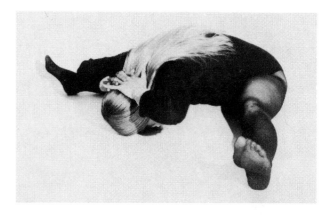

■ The Bow/*Dhanurasana*

The benefits of the Bow posture are greatly increased if you practice
this additional exercise after becoming proficient in the simple positions.

Instead of grasping the ankles, catch hold of your toes, and bend your
legs at the knee so that your heels touch your buttocks [1].

Place your chin on the floor. Your chest, abdomen and thighs are also
on the floor.

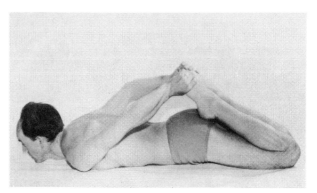

I

Contract the back muscles, and thrust with the abdomen, and your knees and pubic region will rise from the floor [2]. This takes greater muscular effort than the illustration would indicate, the greatest power coming from the arms, while the legs are relaxed. The muscular relationships of this final variant are the direct opposite of those in the normal Bow.

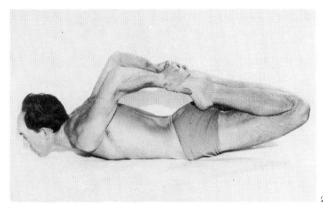

2

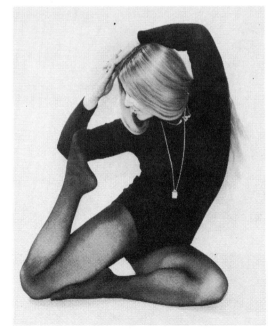

The Pigeon, a pose to promote suppleness and slenderness of the hips.

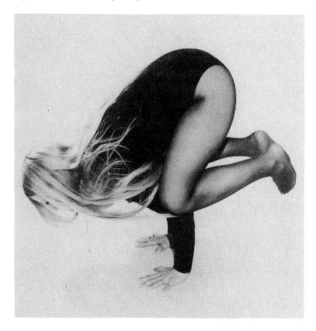

*The Crow and the
Raven need a certain
amount of balance and
strength of arm for
correct performance.
They cannot be held
for any length of time.*

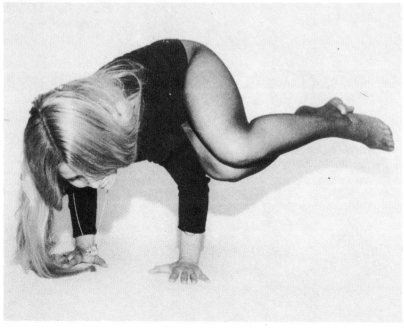

■ Salutation to the Sun/*Suryanamaskar*

It is impossible to contemplate a book of Yoga without including that essential part of Hatha Yoga, the Salutation to the Sun. It comprises, of course, a series of postures and breathing exercises traditionally performed by Yogins daily at Dawn, and forms an excellent morning Eye Openers for those of us who can practice our asanas at other times of the day, or who have the time to perform both the Salutation and the asanas before breakfast. Suryanamaskar takes about ten minutes.

Breathe out, consider the sun as the source of light and of warmth. Consider the light and warmth within yourself [1].

Inhale, raising your arms high and bending backwards at the waist [2]. Consider breath, without which you would die.

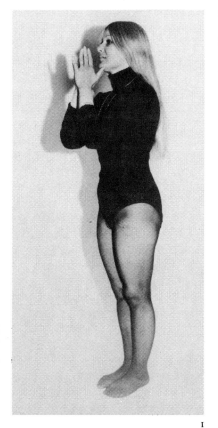

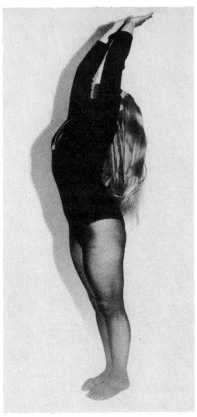

1

2

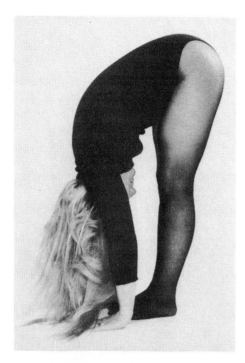

Exhale, bending with straight knees, to touch the floor [3].

Without rising, inhale and extend right leg back, keeping left foot between hands [4].

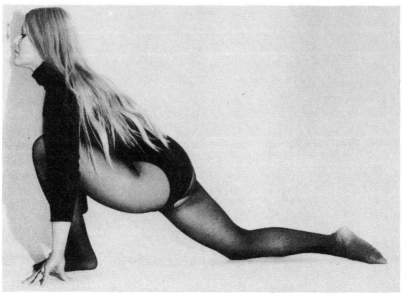

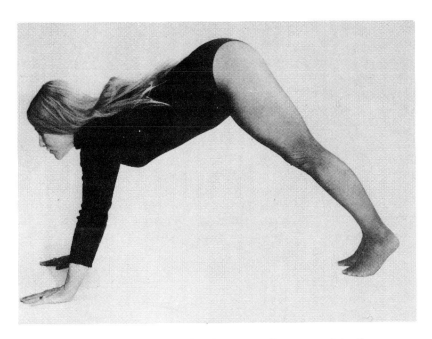

Holding breath, stretch your other leg out to form a straight line between hands and toes [5].

Exhale, rest the body on the ground so that feet, knees, chest, hands and forehead touch the floor, and the pubic region is raised [6].

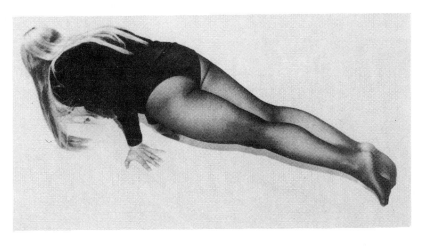

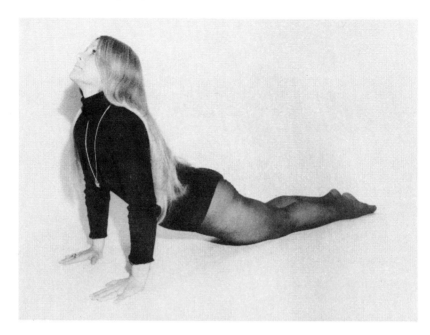

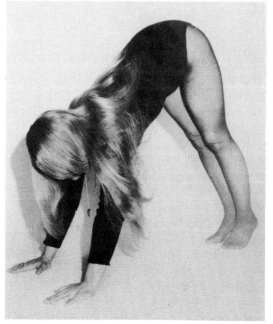

Inhale, pushing chest forward and up, in Cobra position [7].

Exhale, raising hips so that the body forms a triangle [8].

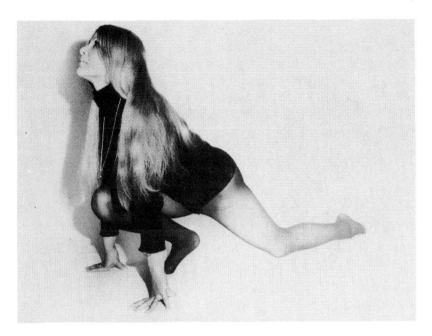

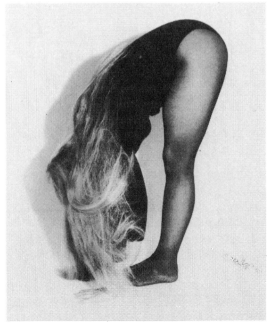

Inhale, and with hands still on the ground, bring right foot forward [9], raising head and arching back, as in position 4.

Exhale, returning to position 3 [10].

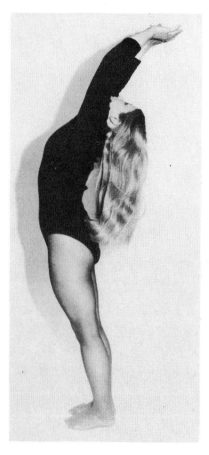 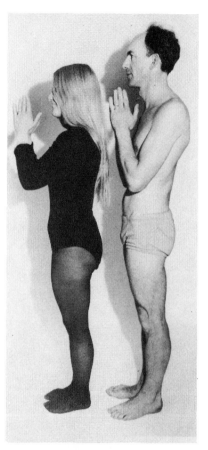

Inhale, assuming position 2 [11].   Exhale, straighten the back, lower
                                       arms [12]. Relax.

Concentration and Meditation

BEFORE we discuss the Yoga exercises in concentration and meditation, it must be made clear that the ultimate goal of the Oriental Yogin is not one which has a great deal of attraction to the average Westerner, who may think it, especially when reading about it, to be irrelevant to his normal daily life. Since this book is designed to be of *practical* benefit to the reader, it may seem to deviate from its practicality at this point, because the ultimate for which the true Eastern Yogin practices concentration and meditation is what is called Samadhi, a state beyond thought, beyond feeling, beyond will, and is the superconsciousness in which his true self is revealed to him. You will find a great many definitions of Samadhi, and none are truly satisfactory. Perhaps, if the words did not have another connotation, one might call it the Moment of Truth.

It is the ultimate in introspection, and therefore is seldom achieved by the basically extrovertive Westerner, but the difficulty in reaching Samadhi does not preclude us from obtaining tremendous personal benefit from the practice of concentration and meditation. Many of the problems of our daily life, and of our own personalities can be very adequately dealt with, and often disappear entirely, as we progress from concentration to meditation. We become less prone to be influenced by other people, or to be bullied or worried by them, and become, as it were, more our own personal property than we ever were before.

Concentration puts our minds in order, and enables us to deal constructively with specific problems. It becomes possible to apply concentration for a few minutes, and to wait for the answer to a problem, or for a new idea which we have vainly seeking simply to come into our mind by the exclusion of all extraneous thoughts.

If this seems an overwhelmingly optimistic promise, something from the realms of magic, one of the three wishes in a fairy tale, it is as well to remember that, before starting the asanas, you probably thought it quite impossible that you could ever stand comfortably on your head, or bend your spine into the Bow. For just as your body learnt to assume what seems to the uninitiated an impossible position, so your mind can learn, by a series of exercises, to respond to a similar kind of control.

Concentration is always preceded by a few rounds of deep breathing.

Concentration Exercises

1] The first exercise that we practice is called *Pratyahara* or sense-withdrawal, in which one becomes as unaware of the world as is possible. Thus, especially in the early stages, one should chose a place in which our senses are as unaware of our surroundings as possible, i.e. our location should be quiet, of even temperature, and, if we prefer it, dark.

If you cannot achieve the Lotus Pose, sit in the cross legged Tailor position, and sit on something neither too hard nor too soft. An Eastern Yogin traditionally sits on a pile of cow hides, which have exactly the right consistancy, but a firm cushion or folded rug is quite adequate. The test of the seat is that you quickly become unaware of it.

Consciously and deliberately 'withdraw' your senses of hearing, sight, smell, breathing deeply. This is easier to actually perform than to describe in words, and even if this control over your senses takes some time to establish, the establishment of it is quite possible, and far easier than you expect. Mental passivity will come with this part of your exercise.

2] As your consciousness of the external world decreases, you can progress to the next stage, which is called *Dharana*, which means the restriction of the mind on a single point. Simply allow thoughts to roam through your mind unchecked, making no attempt to restrict or control them. Detach yourself from your own identity, and monitor the whole proceeding as if you were watching a rather chaotic motion picture.

You may well be surprised, or even shocked, at the thoughts that flow through your mind at this stage, but these are sterile useless emotions, since one cannot always be responsible for what one sees and hears, and thoughts are most often the products of our environment.

As you progress, possibly in your first session, or after two or three, you will find that the chaotic rush of thoughts smooths out to become an orderly chain, with one thought following on after another. Still as an observer of the processes of your own mind, notice how every thought has a beginning, rises to a peak of intensity, and then fades, to be followed by another fulfilling this same pattern.

When each succeeding thought is separated from the thought which preceded it, you can, for a fraction of a second, suppress the arising of your next thought.

This all important fractional pause (which will lengthen with practice), does not result in a 'blank mind', but in your first glimpse of your true self, unhampered by the strictures and stresses of the world, and without the complexes and inhibitions placed upon it from birth. To the Eastern Yogin this pause is the first step on the path to Samadhi, and to the Westerner, it signalizes the beginning of a controlled and ordered mind, and to that knowledge of himself which will help him find his true place in his own particular world.

This is concentration, but it is not concentration *in depth*. This, too, must be learnt, and there in some division among Gurus as to the best method to undertake. If we consider two methods, it is not because we consider one better than another, or that, if one is undertaken, the other should be ignored, but in the recognition that we are all individuals, and may find one method more satisfactory than another.

Visual Concentration

When practising this method, one chooses an object on which to concentrate. (This aids us to think in *pictures*, rather than in words, which can be an inconvenient process of thought, unless our lives are intensely bound up with words. Where our problems deal with the purely practical, or deal with human relationships, visual imagary in thought constitutes an easy and faster language.)

The object chosen can be entirely to our own taste, limited only by our actual physical location at the time of concentration. Thus, outdoors, you might choose a flower or tree, a hill or house in the distance, a river, a road, the sea. Indoors, a picture, an ornament, again a flower, a cup or saucer, a piece of fruit. If you prefer to concentrate in the dark, choose a candle . . . not an electric light bulb, because its light is too strong for a fixed steady gaze. Never concentrate upon the sun, no matter what anyone may tell you. To concentrate properly will certainly damage your sight, possibly permanently.

Once you have chosen your object, place a low stool or table about eighteen inches away from you, so that you will be able to study the object without bending more than your gaze. Your body must remain immobile. If the object is small, hold it in your hand, explore it with your fingers, get to know its shape and texture, its size and weight. Value its imperfections as well as its completeness. If it is fruit or flower, become aware of its scent.

Place the object on the stool or table, and seat yourself comfortably in your pose. Focus your gaze on the object, and consider it further in minute detail. You became familiar with its physical attributes. Now you will think further about it.

If it is an orange, consider where it was grown, how it was cultivated, how it came into your hands via its transport and the greengrocer, its internal structure, the many ways it can be peeled and eaten.

If it is an ornament, consider how it was made, how the colours were laid on, how the light falls upon it, where the shadow lies. If it is an antique, think about the time in which it was made, of the people who may have handled it, of the homes that may have contained it, of its associations in your life.

No matter what object you choose, follow each thought smoothly and easily to its conclusion, excluding all other thoughts without tension or stress (don't *work* at it or you will become tense), and when this becomes impossible, as it well might until you have had practice, gently bring your thoughts back to the object of concentration.

When you have exhausted all the thoughts that you have upon the object (which is not the same thing as all the thoughts there are, by any means), you will no longer be concerned with the shape, size, texture, history of the object, but will hold in your mind the one single idea . . . orange or ornament, candle flame or flower. So completely does the object fill your mind that you become identified with it. You are, at the moment, orange, ornament, candle flame, flower. And in that moment, you have crossed the line between concentration and meditation.

One Point Meditation

Even though we are going to concentrate on an abstract idea, it is often a help until adept to concentrate on a certain portion of the body, such as the point between the eyebrows. (If you have practiced self-awareness, you will already know that such concentration causes a slight but definite sensation in the part which is the subject of the concentration.) This helps to empty the mind for better reception, and there are other techniques, including one which occasionally causes some concern to Westerners . . . the use of the word OM.

We Westerners are probably the only people in the world who can feel embarrassed by actions which we perform in complete privacy, and the thought of sitting cross-legged on the floor solemnly pronouncing the syllable 'OM' would seem to confirm our worse fears about Yoga. Nor are we always reassured when we learn that 'OM' is considered sacred, and that by pronouncing it, we are taking part in a form of worship alien to our own religion.

Actually if we study the meaning of 'OM' we find that it is a symbol of the whole universe, and 'all that is past, present and future . . . and whatever else there is, beyond the threefold divisions of time.' In other words, 'OM' means simply . . . everything, and is a total concept, no matter what religious belief you adhere to. And because of its universality, it makes an ideal subject for meditation.

But there is more to 'OM'. Considered by Oriental philosophers to be the basis of all human sound, the long-drawn-out pronunciation of it will cause the whole of your head to vibrate (to its enormous physical benefit), in a way that no other syllable can equal. If you inhale deeply, and slowly exhale in a prolonged 'Au' sound, you will feel vibrations from the base of your throat to the palate of your mouth, and a hand on your chest will show that these vibrations reach right down to your thoracic cage, massaging nerves and endocrine glands so deeply seated that they are not efficiently reached by the practice of asanas. Closing the mouth and pronouncing a prolonged 'MMMM', you can feel your brain vibrating gently.

The effect of 'OM' is both relaxing and stimulating, and the effect is total, not only being felt throughout the body, but in one's mental reactions, as it reduces depression, and often alleviates feelings of inferiority and other emotional distresses.

There is no other syllable which, repeated, gives such far reaching effects, but every individual is quite at liberty to try to find one. There can be no harmful vibrations from any such sound one can utter, unless one screams at full pitch, in which case one can cause local damage to the vocal cords, and possibly to the ears, if the sound is loud enough.

But one can concentrate and thus pass into meditation without the use of the word 'OM'. Any word which conjures up in our minds a connotation of pleasure will serve. This may be an abstract, such as 'Peace' or 'Truth', or the name of a place with which we have pleasant associations, or even our own names. (Tennyson could evoke what he described as 'a kind of waking trance' from the repetition of his own name.) When we have reached the stage where our minds are filled with no more than an essential idea, we pass from concentration into meditation.

The study of the state of *Dhyana*, the truly meditative stage, is possibly beyond the scope of this book, which is designed to help the average Westerner to cope with the tensions and stresses of an average Western life. The study of Dhyana is intensely interesting, and the practice of it brings us to a full awareness of our essential selves, and of our relationship to the world around us. It is the search for the final basic truths, and continues until death, when it is believed that the final truth will be revealed. One cannot pursue *Dhyana* and remain unchanged, because one's present aims in life become irrelevant, and to a serious seeker after truth, and after Samadhi, a normal life becomes, not so much impracticable, but undesirable.

But to cross the line into meditation during one's concentration exercises is not only desirable, but beneficial, not only because it shows that we have concentrated to the fullest, but because it gives us momentary glimpses of our true selves and of basic truths. Many scientists, including Isaac Newton, found answers to scientific problems when on the edge of the meditative state, and it is possible that a great number of creative people produce their best work when they have, after a period of intense concentration, found a certain 'brain change', a kind of gear change, to a higher state of cerebral acuteness and awareness which leads to a new kind of productivity. This is, perhaps, what we call 'inspiration', which, although it sometimes comes like an intruding flash, is more often the outcome of intense concentration, not necessarily on the subject in hand.

Thus we can benefit directly from both concentration and meditation in dealing with our every day problems. Once we can order our thoughts, and exclude those that are irrelevant, we can really concentrate on and exhaust our thoughts on a single subject. After that, our mind is open to receive that one single clear solution which would otherwise get lost in the crowded hurly-burly of a disordered mind, and the thought is completely ours, because it comes from our real selves, uninfluenced and untrammelled by the tensions placed upon us by other people, and which we unwittingly place upon ourselves.

Once one is practiced in concentration, one can order one's thoughts very quickly, and can practice Pratyahara (sense withdrawal) irrespective of the surroundings. Thus one can face a board meeting, a tricky labour situation, the creation of yet another pithy copy headline, the presentation of a costing programme with a mind wholly focussed on the job in hand, without any fear of interruption from external sources, or from within one's own head. You are in control of yourself and of the situation, and if you are inclined to be dominated by other people against your better judgement, this will be overcome, because so well marshalled are your thoughts that you will know precisely why you believe another's judgements to be faulty. You are, in fact, totally 'clear headed'.

But this doesn't come in a day. Let's concentrate on the orange, 'OM' or our own name first. And remember our Yoga breathing.

Yoga Hygiene

THOSE of us who have travelled in Eastern countries, particularly during war-time, may not be impressed by the general hygienic standards of the Oriental races, but we cannot tell which individuals, among the milling millions, are Yogins, nor can we be aware of their habits and personal cleanliness. since they are performed in private. Thus we Westerners should not reject the example of the few simply because we consider our way of life to be superior to the many.

There are a number of hygienic procedures carried out by Eastern Yogins from a very early age under the direction of a Guru (teacher) from the time they first become disciples. Many of these procedures are described in popular books on Yoga, but carry certain dangers to the uninitiated, especially when working without expert guidance, and should the reader come across them, he is advised to treat them as being of academic interest only.

But the study of Yoga introduces one to completely new thinking on the matter of personal hygiene, and this follows, not by any rule or law in the Yoga way of life, but simply from the fact that, if one practices self-awareness, it becomes slightly disgusting to be aware of a body that is not as clean as it might be.

This awareness leads one deeper than the normal civilized practices of bathing, hair-washing, tooth-cleaning and toe-nail-cutting, because in becoming aware of our internal organs, we become aware of, not only their functions, but of their disfunctions and the abuses to which we subject them.

As we practise self-awareness, and think, in turn, of our internal organs, we cannot but think of their functions in the maintenance of our bodies, of the use to which they are put, and whether these uses are to their benefit or not. In contemplating our digestive systems, we automatically think of the food we put into our stomachs, and the effect of that food, particularly on the liver. Those of us who would not dream of using too rich a mixture in a motor scooter, or too high an octane of petrol in our car often cram our digestions with fatty foods and alcohol, to the detriment of our livers and gall bladders.

You may wonder why this aspect of self-awareness is being dealt with in a chapter on hygiene, but it will be self-evident that, if the external cleanliness which we normally practice is largely a matter of self respect, the proper cleansing of our internal organs is a monitor of our own good health. Most of us have known at some time the vague ill-health of biliousness or constipation, and have resorted to a liver pill or laxative to offset what we unfortunately consider the normal penalties of everyday living.

It is virtually impossible to separate one aspect of Yoga from another, since it represents a total way of life, and although we do not follow the rather stringent bodily routines of the Oriental Yogins to clear stomach and bowels, we soon find that the Yoga Diet and the asanas will cure the most obstinate and chronic constipation, and the massage and decongestion of liver and gall bladder stimulate these organs to perform their functions correctly. In actual fact, liver pills and laxatives, while providing temporary relief by cathartic action, by this very action create a repetition of the condition they are said to cure. There is no physical law that dictates that every human individual must have a daily bowel movement, and if you discontinue the laxative habit and follow a sensible moderate diet, your digestive system will soon establish its natural rhythm to the general benefit of your health. If you wish to avoid a bilious liver, you must allow it to function within its own limitations of efficiency. If you constantly overload it with rich fatty foods and alcohol, you cannot expect it to heal itself by means of a pill which is almost purely laxative, anyway, and if you subject it to an increased stimulation of bile, you must expect it to need rest, and it will be less able to deal with over-indulgences following its harsh treatment.

Thus, if one respects one's body, one must treat it, not only with respect, but with reasonable commonsense, not putting into one's mouth more than can be efficiently dealt with by one's digestive and aliminatory systems. If we consider our bodies to be the vehicles of our progression through life, we should not subject them to less care or less reasonable usage than we would give a car, a watch or a combined harvester.

Yoga disciplines are personal, and if we submit to them, it is because we as individuals decide that we should. Yogins are not *forced* to abstain from eating or drinking unwisely, or to perform the asanas, or to practice the systems of Yoga hygiene. There is no club from which you can be expelled for breaking the rules. Nobody will pass a vote of censure on you, there is no breathaliser test, no secret police will knock on your door at night. Every single action you take, or decision you make with regard to anything in the Yoga way of life is between you and yourself, and an entirely personal matter.

But as you lie relaxed on the floor, and practice self-awareness, it becomes impossible, when you really make the acquaintance of your internal organs, as well as the rest of your anatomy, to contemplate the fact that your skin could be dirty, your digestive tract crammed with unnecessary detritus, your liver eroded, your teeth decayed, your tongue furred, your stomach inflamed, and your lungs only partly active, and (if you are a smoker) filled with phlegm and tar deposits.

This may be the first time in your life that you have come to the full realisation of the damage that 'life', in its purely personal terms, can inflict upon your bodies. Most of us automatically resist external pressures to take up this and that, and to give up this and that, and our resistance is a manifestation of our own desire for personal liberty. It is only when we apply our own disciplines that we can do so without mental block, and can be sure of success.

We have already said that many of the hygienic techniques practiced by Oriental Yogins are not suitable for Westerners, but there are two Yoga habits of cleanliness which we might adopt with great advantage.

The first is called 'Neti', a form of nasal douche, and is, incidentally, a very effective way of avoiding a cold or curing an existing one. We are often advised to 'sniff up salt water' as cure or preventative, but when one tries it, one comes to the conclusion that the adviser must either have a special technique, or is acting in a spirit of revenge, because one seldom gets past the first sniff without choking, and ends up with a partially cleaned nose, and a raw throat into the bargain.

The reason for this is because a sniff is a comparatively violent action in a region very sensitive to violence. The water goes up the nostril far too far and far too fast, producing a drowning sensation, and if we choke, it is more from this reason than from the amount of water we swallow.

However, the basic principle is sound, and we will make use of it, simply as a basic principle. We fill a small bowl with tepid water, and add a teaspoon of salt.

We are going to pump the water up the nostrils by means of a pumping mechanism most of us have never realised that we possess. You can make tiny movements at the back of your throat, and if you find it difficult at first, practice, head *out* of water, by repeating a hard G sound right at the back of the throat. Not the phonetic G, but G as in gate or garden. When one closes one's mouth, the sound becomes impossible to make, and one simply makes pumping movements at the back of the throat, which sounds like water pouring from a narrow-necked bottle, or running down a drain pipe.

To perform Neti, one covers one's nostrils with the tepid salted water simply by dipping in one's nose, and pumps away, and if the water is at the correct temperature (the standard test is to dip one's elbow into it), one is unaware of the water entering until one tastes the salt as the water enters the throat.

Stop pumping, and hold the breath for a few seconds, nose still in the water, and then raise the head and allow the water to run out of the nose. Repeat the whole operation twice.

Finish the exercise by blocking one nostril and exhaling vigorously through the other, to dispel the remains of the water. Repeat with the other nostril. Your nasal passages should be completely clear, and in addition, the nerve-endings of your aural cavity should have been stimulated to the extent that you immediately find an improvement in your senses of smell and sight.

The technique of exhaling through one nostril while blocking the other has another application in our normal hygienic practices, even if it can only be confined to the bathroom for aesthetic reasons. Physiologically it is a far safer and more effective practice than the ordinary blowing of the nose, and is more likely to completely clear the nasal passages. Vigorous nose blowing can damage the delicate nasal tissues, and can cause distention of the veins.

In the chapter of Yoga Breathing, we mentioned the practice of the Cleansing Breath (Kapalabhati), and although it makes a good start to a round of breathing exercises, it also has its place in the daily hygiene routine, and is therefore included in this chapter.

To perform the Cleansing Breath, take a deep breath, filling your lungs completely, and exhale in short sharp puffs, aided by quick inward jerks of the abdominal muscles and the diaphragm. This will clear the nasal passages and sinuses extremely effectively. Continue these sharp exhalations until the lungs are empty, and then inhale again.

There are several basic differences between the Cleansing Breath and other breathing exercises, insofar as in this case, the exhalation time is shorter than that of inhalation, and the breath is not held between inhalation and exhalation. A pause follows a round of ten inhalation/exhalations, and should consist of about a minute's normal breathing. Further rounds can follow as you feel inclined.

Another difference . . . the efficiency of the exercise lies in the speed of the sharp short exhalations, and in the number that you can cram in before the air in your lungs is exhausted. You should be able to manage two exhalations per second, but it is a mistake to concentrate on speed and timing at the expense of the strong inward abdominal stroke which gives the required force to your exhalations.

If you perform your exercise correctly, you may expect some soreness in your abdominal muscles until they become attuned to the quick forceful action, but this will pass comparatively quickly, especially as the practice of the asanas will strengthen your muscles.

The final hygienic practice is called Tongue Dhauti (Dhauti simply means 'a purification practice') and is concerned with the cleansing of this much neglected organ. Those of us who clean our teeth as a matter of automatic habit seldom stop to think that whatever is capable of clinging to our teeth can also cling to our tongue, and with far more reaching effect.

The tongue is considerably concerned with eating, and with the digestion of our food. It acts as a kind of flexible paddle which churns the food around in our mouths to soften it. It is a prime-mover in the action of swallowing. It is covered with taste buds, which not only enable us to enjoy our food (and to distinguish good food from bad), but which actually assist in the stimulation of the secretion of ptyalin, the first digestive fluid encountered in the digestive system. Think how, when you are ill or over-tired, and force yourself to eat food you don't particularly want (an ill-advised practice at the best of times), the food remains dry and hard in your mouth, and simply won't soften, because your taste buds have temporarily gone out of action, and there is no digestive stimulation.

If you take a critical look at your tongue, and the chances are that you will wonder how your taste buds ever function at all, because few of us seem to be able to present a pink clean healthy tongue for our own inspection. (The Western idea that the state of our tongue reflects the state of our liver is only partly correct, as the practice of Tongue Dhauti will show. However, over-indulgence does show itself in a furry tongue, as most of us know from personal experience.)

Eastern Yogins cleanse their tongues with special wooden scrapers, but the handy Western equivalent is a coffee spoon or small teaspoon. Simply scrape the tongue with the edges of the bowl of the spoon, and one glance at the result will convince you, not only that you should continue the exercise until no more detritus can be removed, but to repeat it henceforward at regular intervals. You will, in fact, be amazed!

Some people are inclined to 'gag' when their tongues are touched, possibly because they were victims in childhood of the use of tongue depressors when their throats were examined. This effect is minimized or disappear completely when the tongue is scraped *across* its surface, and not along it, and if one takes this sideways scraping further back at each session, the gagging disappears.

You may feel inclined to ask whether it would not be better to brush the tongue in the same way as the teeth, possibly using tooth paste or powder, but there are two dangers in this practice. First, the tongue is a fairly delicate organ which may be scored by the bristles of the brush (and dentifrices are scouring agents), and secondly, tooth brushing is a relatively clumsy operation. Working in the dark, as it were, it is quite possible to damage the soft palate with the head of the brush, and this is a very delicate organ indeed, and its repair unpleasant, to say the least.

The direct result of Tongue Dhauti, outside of the aesthetic effect of being able to contemplate its cleanliness during your Self Awareness exercise, is the fact that your sense of taste becomes almost immediately far keener, enabling you to enjoy your food far more. This in turn stimulates the first stages of digestion, giving your food a good start on its journey through the digestive tract. It is, in fact, a considerable bonus to be obtained for the price of a coffee spoon and an occasional extra few minutes added to your normal toilet routine.

Yoga Diet . . . a New Look at Food

ECAUSE YOGA is a total way of life, dietary rules were laid down early for its followers, and because Yoga was originally exclusive to the East, the diet was completely suitable to the Oriental. Buddhists eat no meat, because it is against their religion to take life, for food or for any other reason. Hindus normally eat meat, but Hindu Yogins do not, because the prohibitions against taking life extends to all who follow the Yoga Way of Life, not only to the Buddhists.

But although most Yogins are vegetarians, this is not a plea for vegetarianism, which is always a matter of personal taste, and above all, not a plea for *instant* vegetarianism, since the sudden introduction of any radically new diet can cause as sudden a stomach upset.

The perfect Yoga diet of the Oriental Yogin included moderation and a certain amount of abstension within a regimen which was, because of widespread poverty, already abstemious in the extreme. The average Westerner would hardly have been able to survive on the normal diet, even before the Yoga aesthetes pared it away by eating less, and even simpler food.

However, in admitting that the true Yoga diet is unsuitable for the Westerner, we have to recognise the fact that our own present day diet is itself by no means ideal, because, by custom, we not only eat too much, not only eat the wrong foods, but often eat too much of the wrong foods.

Today's food, as we all know, is not what it used to be, viewed from any nutritional standard ever devised. Not only has a great deal of its value been removed from our daily food, often to be replaced chemically, but almost all the food we buy has been processed or frozen before it reaches us, or contains some kind of preservative.

If food is not what it was, neither is it always what it appears to be. Few people read the wording on packages, although it often makes very interesting reading, and even fewer people are aware, for instance, that they eat artificial protein in such convenient foods as beef curry and certain types of Chinese foods. This artificial protein may eventually save the world from starvation, but its very existence, often unsuspected, makes us wonder exactly how much we know about the food we eat. It is only when some 'scare', as in the case of cyclamates, makes newspaper headlines that we become aware of our own ignorance in this vital matter.

We do not need reminding that incorrect diet (incorrect in both quantity and content), can cause as many conditions of ill-health as can the tensions of modern living. Many of us force ourselves to read the warning articles in the Press, and we often decide, at some time, to follow a safer and more beneficial plan of eating, for our own protection. This resolution usually goes by default the next time we enter a restaurant, snatch a hurried office lunch, or help ourselves through a boring day with a cup of coffee and a cream cake.

It isn't easy to depart from what we know to be an unfortunate eating plan, since ninety percent of the population of the Western world eat denatured over-rich convenience foods, and most of the products on the market are directed to this ninety percent. It is an unfortunate fact that, if we want our food to reach us in its natural state we must pay more for it, and search for it into the bargain. But, as we explain later in this chapter, we will find ourselves wanting to eat less, which will compensate for the slight extra cost, and the small amount of extra trouble, involved in eating for perfect health, and there are a great many ways in which we can improve our general nutritional picture without radically altering our present way of life.

Even if we are not going to adopt the rigid Yoga diet, there are certain tenets of Yoga with regard to eating which will improve your health a great deal, even before you change your diet.

1] Since the Yoga philosophy is always concerned with moderation, Yogins are exhorted to eat moderately, to leave one quarter of their stomach empty, and never to be conscious of a feeling of fullness. The slight feeling of hunger that you experience at first in eating smaller sized meals, will soon disappear. The stomach is an accommodating organ, and just as it accommodates itself now to a larger meal than is required, so it will learn to contract when presented with smaller meals, and hunger will no longer be felt.

2] If we eat less, we should make maximum use of the food that we do eat. Yogins place great importance on the complete chewing of each mouthful of food, so that the first stage of the digestive process can be properly completed before swallowing, and maximum absorption can take place in the digestive tract, which does not happen if food is swallowed improperly chewed.

Gladstone, who chewed every mouthful of milk pudding thirty-two times, obeyed this sensible principle, but must be accounted a monumental bore for this fact to have become universally known. To count one's jaw movements is to give far too much importance to a minor routine in one's life. Properly masticated food attains a soft paste-like consistency, and slips easily down the gullet, and this is the only criterion we need.

While benefiting from these two important points, we can also consider an easy stage-by-stage plan towards a healthier diet. In suggesting weekly stages, we are, of course, aware that the ultimate benefits can be achieved quicker if the process were speeded up. This, of course, is a personal matter, as so much in the Yoga philosophy is a personal matter, and if you, as an individual, tend to resist change, the weekly plan may be easier for you.

First Week

1] Discontinue the use of refined white sugar, and use raw (brown) sugar instead. Demarara sugar adds no 'treacly' taste to tea or coffee. Avoid sweets, jams and other products containing white sugar, substituting honey, which can also be used to sweeten puddings. Hot milk and honey makes an excellent bed-time drink, as it induces sleep.

2] Switch from white bread to brown, and avoid, as far as possible, white flour products.

Second Week

1] Continue as above.

2] Discontinue the use of chemical salt, and substitute sea salt. (Most good quality grocers stock it. Health Food Shops certainly do.)

3] Avoid pepper and other hot spices. (Herbs are not prohibited.)

4] Substitute milk or fruit juice for one or more of your daily cups of tea or coffee.

Third Week

1] Continue as above.

2] Try a Meusli breakfast. The combination of cereal, dried fruit and nuts, with milk, will give you a full nutritional picture on which to start the day.

3] Avoid all meat products containing preservative, e.g. sausages of all kinds, butcher's mince, packaged hamburgers etc.

4] Substitute fresh fruit for puddings a few days a week.

Fourth Week

1] Continue as above.

2] Reduce the amount of meat eaten at any meal by eating extra vegetables and salads.

3] Reduce the number of meat meals eaten, substituting cheese or egg dishes.

4] Increase consumption of milk or fruit juice as a substitute for tea or coffee.

5] Reduce the amount of fried foods eaten. Grill or dry-roast in foil, as an alternative to frying.

Such a diet need not be dull. You can do more with fresh fruit than bring it to the table unpeeled. Furit sorbets and granitas are a delicious substitute for commercially made ice creams. It is possible to obtain endless permutations and combinations in fresh fruit salad, and as your sense of taste improves, you will be able to enjoy them even more.

Fruit and cheese naturally go together, not only the usual apples and Cheddar, but pears, grapes and fresh pineapple with almost any cheese.

But it is up to you to find your own favourite combination, and the cheese board and fruit bowl together make a second course which outclasses almost any dessert you might like to name.

If up to this moment you have considered vegetables and salads dull, it might be worth mentioning that there are many things you can do with vegetables besides boiling them to death with a pinch of bicarbonate of soda. And there are many good salads that go beyond a slice each of tomato and beetroot on a lettuce leaf. A new look at food presupposes a new look at cooking and preparation, too, and there are plenty of good cookery books with ideas you may not have thought of.

It is relatively easy to implement a new eating plan within one's own home, but eating out sometimes presents problems. It is said, with sad truth, that there is no bore like a diet bore, and none of us likes to be considered 'faddy', or part of one of the many lunatic fringes on the edge of what is commonly called normal society. To go to a dinner party and refuse to eat half the meal because of one's dietary prohibitions, classes one not only as a bore, but as a discourteous bore, and to be known as a food faddist in advance of a dinner party (our reputation having proceeded us), will not only throw our hostess into a panic, but ensure that we are dropped from further invitation lists. Good manners dictate that we should eat and enjoy (or give every appearance of enjoying) the meals that are served to us, and nothing makes us social outcasts as fast as picking at food which has been carefully selected, prepared and served.

But by the time you have reached the fourth week of your diet plan, you will also have reached the fourth week of your Yoga asanas, and will be well on the way to becoming a new individual. You will be healthier, your colour and complexion will be better, you will have improved posture and more poise, and will certainly have lost weight if you needed to. A certain amount of food selection will be granted you on these grounds alone, because people are invariably prone to consider any visible improvement in health, especially where loss of weight is concerned, as being solely due to diet.

If your future hostess phones you, her voice quivering with apprehension, to say that she has heard you have taken up some new diet, and to ask what you can or cannot eat, it is quite sufficient to say that your diet is quite ordinary, except that you don't eat as much meat as you used to, so that a small slice would be sufficient, because you eat more vegetables, fruit and cheese. This enables her to go ahead with

her plans, and to put on a cheese board, which she would probably
do anyway. If she does not ask for prior information, you can follow
this plan without discourtesy, and it is a relatively small matter,
anyway, unless you dine out every day of the week. An occasional meal
outside your prescribed diet does little damage, as long as you remember
that you are now eating less, and proper chewing will ensure that you
do not finish your meal ahead of the 'bolters' who are eating more.

In Yoga, you will find that food tends to assume its proper place in
your life, in that it is no longer given an exaggerated importance. This
does not mean that you cease to enjoy your meals, in fact, you develop
a keener sense of taste and enjoy them more, but the chances are that
you won't need any force of will to eat less . . . you simply won't feel
that you need the quantity of food that you previously did. And once
you find your tensions disappearing, you find that you no longer need
to reward yourself with food (this being commonly the result of tension),
or to eat to relieve boredom. This is easier to experience than to
describe, but is common to most Yogins. One can also avoid feeling
hungry when eating would be inconvenient once one has built up a
certain measure of bodily control.

This might be a good time, since we have been discussing dinner
parties, to raise the question of alcohol. Under the Yoga rules, no
Eastern Yogin drinks or smokes, but when we are not contemplating
the complete aesthetic way of life, this is again a purely personal
matter. There are constant social pressures on most of us to drink
alcohol, and one often hesitates to take a personal stand on this matter,
for fear of ridicule, or of being accused of taking up a 'Holier than
Thou' attitude. And, let's face it, most of us like to take a drink, and
enjoy the effects produced by a moderate amount of alcohol.

Alcohol has a liberating effect on many of us, removing tensions and
inhibitions, and we often drink for this very reason. It begets a mild
amnesia, too, and is often the only way that we can lay down the
burdens of our present life for a few minutes. If this is our only reason
for drinking, we will no longer need it, because our concentration and
meditation exercises will enable us to do all these things without a
single drink, because we can not only forget our problems for as long
as we want to, but are enabled to tackle them and overcome them,
so that the underlying cause of our tension is removed.

Where drinking is a real problem, Yoga can be an inestimable help,
because as we learn that the mind can control the body (the first lesson
being concentration during asanas, which makes smooth movement

very much easier), we also learn that we can control the impulses
of the body and the thoughts of the mind. Thus, instead of making
mind and body a constant battlefield in a war against alcoholism, we
can create periods during meditation when the thoughts of taking a
drink do not exist. If these periods are fractional at first, they can be
lengthened with practice, and teach us, if nothing else, that there are
periods in our life when alcohol is not important. In creating a non-
alcoholic 'corner' in our lives, we break at least a few bars of the iron
cage that encloses us, and makes us realise that it might, after all, be
possible for us to cure ourselves.

Alcoholism is now accepted as a disease, and just as the arthritic will
find bodily relief in the judicious practice of asanas to loosen tightened
joints, so the alcoholic will find great physical benefit from the
exercises, especially in increased blood circulation and in the massage
of internal organs. A stage is reached, and reached very soon after
taking up Yoga, when a person suffering from *any* progressive physical
condition will say 'This is not something that I want to happen to my
body, because it is not only inconvenient, it is also disrespectful.'
The physical benefits of Hatha Yoga are not gratuitious by-products of
a set of exercises performed for some esoteric reason. Since they were
designed to produce these benefits, and since they create a state of
maximum health, there is hardly a physical state that does not improve
under their regimen.

The greatest lesson that we can learn from Yoga with regard to
alcoholism and hard-line smoking is that we do not have to indulge in
a *battle* to overcome them. To engage in a battle indicates that the
battle can be lost, but passive action can be easy and gradual and
cannot be defeated. Since both these problems are partly physical,
the asanas help us to rid ourselves of these physical effects far quicker
than any other routine of exercises. Since we quickly reach the stage
in either smoking or drinking (or both), where abstinence causes tension
which is added to the deeply underlying tension which probably
caused us to drink or smoke in the first place, we can, almost as
quickly lose them by the practice of the asanas and by relaxation
exercises, and drive them further away by sessions of meditation. Those
of us who are not plagued by either of these problems cannot realise
the importance of a fractional pause (which will grow longer in
time), in a life of endless craving for a cigarette or drink, and few
of those with these problems will have much faith, until they have tried
it, in the ability of Yoga to help them control mind and body so that

the disease becomes on a par with any other, to be lessened as health improves, and to become under the control of the will as the exercises in meditation progress. If one reads the chapter on Yoga Hygiene and self-awareness, one readily sees the virtual impossibility of wanting to flood the blood with alcohol, or of constantly drawing smoke into our lungs.

But in the discovery that alcoholism and hard-line smoking are diseases, we have possibly unwittingly put too much emphasis upon them, with ill-effects upon those who suffer from them. The body is, after all, only one-third of our total entity, and is simply the machine which enables us to progress through life. We maintain it in good health the better to live the lives of our minds and spirits, and if we consider it in this light, it becomes only good sense not to abuse it. This is simple logic, but we humans are not particularly logical. We fear death, and yet hasten it in almost every conceivable way by the very life that we have created, by tension, by inaction, by a thousand abuses accepted by us as part of our way of life, so that at the end of it, we may well ask ourselves, 'What happened? Where did Life go?

It is far better to be able to say, 'I know the answer. I was aware of Life. I made the best of what I was given.'

Summary of Asanas

Asana	Effect	Benefits	Contra indications
Shoulder Stand	Reverse position	Increase circulation, especially to the brain. Stretches spine, also leg, back, abdominal muscles. Tones nervous system, Rejuvination, weight reduction. Benefits all glands, especially thyroid.	Do not attempt the asana in casesof cerebral sclerosis, severe otitis or sinusitis, angina.
Plough	Backward spinal stretch	Promotes suppleness of spine and of almost all muscles. Improves circulation, especially of spine. Tones nervous system, helps correct spinal curvature. Rejuvination, weight reduction.	Hernia First days of menstrual cycle.
Fish	Spinal arch (Countering the action of the plough.)	Promotes suppleness of spine and thorax, the latter with great benefit to the lungs. Removes stiffness in upper spine and neck, improves posture, corrects spinal curvature, strengthens back muscles, improves circulation, massages internal organs.	
Forward Bend	Posterior spinal Stretch	Stretches muscles of back, abdomen, arms, legs. Tones all internal organs, and upper region of the spine. Separates each vertebra to release spinal nerves. Reduces hips and thighs, flattens stomach by strengthening abdominal muscles. Aids digestion, cures chronic constipation.	

Asana	*Effect*	*Benefits*	*Contra indications*
Cobra	Backward spinal stretch	Promotes suppleness of spine and efficiency of nervous system, stretching muscles of abdomen, back, arms and neck, increasing their strength. Regulates body metabolism by thyroid action, massages all internal organs, aids chest expansion. Improves posture, corrects round shoulders.	Spinal pain, not to be confused with natural stiffness when the exercise is first attempted.
Locust	Pelvic lift	Increases flexibility and muscular strength in lumbar spine, guarding against 'weak back' conditions. Tones nerves of lower body, massages internal organs, especially kidneys, increases circulation, corrects spinal curvature.	
Bow	Backward spinal stretch	Promotes spinal flexibility, increased lung capacity and efficiency of all internal organs. Tones muscles of abdomen, back, legs, arms and neck. Combats cellulitis, rheumatism, and lassitude. May help sufferers from Diabetes Mellitus by stimulating pancreatic action. Combats chronic constipation. Creates great feeling of wellbeing.	
Twist	Spinal twist, first one way, and then the other	Benefit to spinal column, nerves, blood vessels is *total*. The action prevents fusing of lower spine, considered a normal 'ageing process'. Internal organs are massaged by compression. Prevents development of lumbago and other back ailments.	
Head Stand	Reverse position	Effects similar to those of the Shoulder Stand, with greatly increased benefits of relaxation and concentration, also rejuvination, often banishing wrinkles and grey hair. Increases intellectual capacity, improves sight and hearing. Often relieves headaches, may help migraine sufferers. Aids treatment of varicose veins and haemorrhoids. (Treatment should be continued nevertheless.) Sufferers from astigmatism, myopia etc. may benefit greatly from this exercise.	Such eye conditions as detached retina, glaucoma, severe conjunctivitis.